D0891199

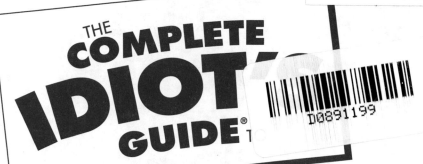

Fitness Boxing

Illustrated

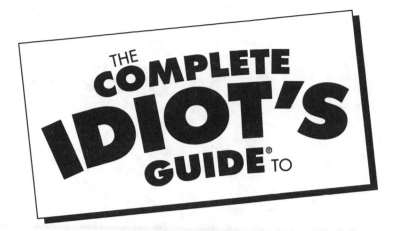

Fitness Boxing

Illustrated

by Tom Seabourne, Ph.D.

ALPHA

A member of Penguin Group (USA) Inc.

I would like to dedicate this book to my friends and sparring partners: Ernest Herndon, Vance McLaughlin, Mike Martin, and Raymond McCallum.

ALPHA BOOKS

Published by the Penguin Group

Penguin Group (USA) Inc., 375 Hudson Street, New York, New York 10014, U.S.A.

Penguin Group (Canada), 10 Alcorn Avenue, Toronto, Ontario, Canada M4V 3B2 (a division of Pearson Penguin Canada Inc.)

Penguin Books Ltd., 80 Strand, London WC2R 0RL, England

Penguin Ireland, 25 St Stephen's Green, Dublin 2, Ireland (a division of Penguin Books Ltd.)

Penguin Group (Australia), 250 Camberwell Road, Camberwell, Victoria 3124, Australia (a division of Pearson Australia Group Pty. Ltd.)

Penguin Books India Pvt. Ltd., 11 Community Centre, Panchsheel Park, New Delhi—110 017, India

Penguin Group (NZ), cnr Airborne and Rosedale Roads, Albany, Auckland 1310, New Zealand (a division of Pearson New Zealand Ltd.)

Penguin Books (South Africa) (Pty.) Ltd., 24 Sturdee Avenue, Rosebank, Johannesburg 2196, South Africa

Penguin Books Ltd., Registered Offices: 80 Strand, London WC2R 0RL, England

International Standard Book Number: 1-59257-503-x
Library of Congress Catalog Card Number: 2005938294

08 07 06   8 7 6 5 4 3 2 1

Interpretation of the printing code: The rightmost number of the first series of numbers is the year of the book's printing; the rightmost number of the second series of numbers is the number of the book's printing. For example, a printing code of 06-1 shows that the first printing occurred in 2006.

Printed in the United States of America

Publisher: *Marie Butler-Knight*
Editorial Director: *Mike Sanders*
Acquisitions Editor: *Paul Dinas*
Managing Editor: *Billy Fields*
Development Editor: *Lynn Northrup*
Copy Editor: *Tricia Liebig*

Cartoonist: *Richard King*
Cover Designer: *Becky Harmon*
Book Designers: *Trina Wurst/Kurt Owens*
Indexer: *Tonya Heard*
Layout: *Becky Harmon*
Proofreading: *Mary Hunt*

Contents at a Glance

Contents

Foreword

People have known since the ancient Greeks that exercise and physical activity are essential to a healthful and productive life. Modern society and the associated sedentary lifestyles have led to a life that requires very little exercise or physical activity. Now people have to design and build exercise and physical activity into their lifestyles, which takes knowledge, motivation, and long-term commitment. You are probably considering *The Complete Idiot's Guide to Fitness Boxing Illustrated* because you want to look and feel better, which means you want to be healthier. You know you need the knowledge, motivation, and long-term commitment, and Tom Seabourne's book provides the tools to become knowledgeable, motivated, and committed.

Typically, a health and fitness instructor (like me) is interested in improving the health-related fitness, which is cardiorespiratory fitness, body composition (percent body fat), muscular strength, muscular endurance, and flexibility of our students or clients. The program presented by Tom Seabourne certainly would allow you to improve and maintain your health-related fitness. But fitness boxing will produce additional fitness benefits in relation to improved balance, coordination, and agility. Exercise or physical activity in a variety of forms has been shown to relieve anxiety and prevent distress. Fitness boxing with imaginary opponents truly gives you the chance to let off some "steam" with an activity that allows you to be physically aggressive without hurting anyone or getting hurt. Fitness boxing is a fun way to get and stay in condition for a healthier life.

If exercise is healthful, why are so many people sedentary or physically inactive? People cite two primary reasons: "exercise is not fun" and "lack of time." Fitness boxing, as presented by Tom Seabourne, deals with those two barriers. If you follow the fitness boxing program, it is fun. There is a tremendous amount of flexibility in terms of time and locations associated with the program. You can be a member of class in a fitness club or you can do mini-workouts in your office. You can use the program as your total fitness program or as part of your exercise regimen. You are in control and make the decisions on the fitness boxing path you will take.

In selecting any book or program, the reader should have two main questions. Is the author qualified? Is the book written and presented in a style that will be entertaining and informative? In the arena of health and exercise, Tom Seabourne has done it all. I can think of no author better qualified to present fitness boxing. The book is presented in a "fun" manner with many supporting features that truly make for a foolproof learning and personal development experience.

—Allen W. Jackson, EdD, FACSM, FAAKPE
Regents Professor
University of North Texas

Introduction

Fitness boxing workouts were inspired by the *Rocky* movies, but Hilary Swank's Oscar-winning performance in the 2004 film *Million Dollar Baby* brought the moves to new generations of fitness enthusiasts searching for workouts that deliver results and ignited a fitness explosion.

Fitness boxing delivers a total-body workout and you don't need to join a gym to learn to bob-and-weave. No sparring partner is necessary, and the equipment requirements are minimal—a bag, wraps, gloves, jump rope, timer, and music. You train like a boxer except you never get hit. But you don't have to step into the ring to get a great workout.

The Complete Idiot's Guide to Fitness Boxing Illustrated brings you the best workouts from the most highly conditioned boxers in the world. It teaches you how to train like a boxer and get all the benefits from doing so. You'll learn how to do great, full-body workouts that are safe, intense, fun, and, best of all, that will put you in the best shape of your life.

Fitness boxing works your whole body in every way imaginable. You improve your heart's function, increase your speed, reaction time, and agility. You train at your own pace increasing your stamina, energy, and concentration.

Because boxing uses muscles in your lower legs, upper legs, buns, waist, chest, shoulders, and arms, you burn more calories than other forms of exercise. A typical boxing workout burns up to 900 calories an hour.

Fat loss isn't the only advantage. You improve your balance with our fancy footwork drills, release stress, improve your cardiovascular fitness, and increase your metabolism. You also firm muscle, develop eye-hand-foot coordination, and elevate your self-confidence—all while having a great time.

The Complete Idiot's Guide to Fitness Boxing Illustrated is a great workout for all fitness levels. It gives you the tools to contour your physique according to your goals. Each chapter progresses from the simplest to the most advanced moves. If you need a recipe for building strength, read the chapter on heavy bag training. To slim down, follow the directions in the footwork chapter. Combine all the drills in all the chapters to get in the best shape of your life.

What You'll Find in This Book

The Complete Idiot's Guide to Fitness Boxing Illustrated is a step-by-step program with more than 200 photographs of easy-to-follow exercises. Begin with a good warm up, learn stances and movement drills, perform defensive tactics, throw combination punches, shadowbox, execute footwork patterns, hit the bag, and then cool down. There you have it—one of the quickest fat-burning, muscle-toning circuit workouts in existence.

The information is divided into four parts:

Part 1, "Getting Ready to Rumble," introduces you to fitness boxing and gives you the foundation to make your commitment to the program.

Part 2, "Building a Boxer's Body," teaches you how to use various equipment to enhance your workouts, tells you what to expect from fitness boxing classes, and introduces partner drills.

By the time you get to **Part 3, "Becoming a Contender,"** you'll probably realize that boxing isn't as easy as it looks. This part breaks it all down and shows you tons of drills that will teach you how to move with grace and power.

Part 4, "Going the Distance," begins with one of the best tools for getting and staying in shape. You'll also learn partner drills that will kick your workouts up a notch, and cool downs and stretches that will prepare you for the next round.

Throughout this book you'll also find four types of sidebars that offer additional insights, definitions, cautions, and other information:

Clear as a Bell _____

In these boxes you'll find definitions of boxing and fitness boxing terms and concepts.

Corner Man _____

These boxes offer quick tips on performing fitness boxing exercises correctly and keeping good form.

Knockout Punch _____

Check these boxes for moves to avoid and other advice on staying healthy and injury-free.

Sweet Science _____

Here you'll find information and insights on boxing and fitness boxing exercises.

Acknowledgments

First I would like to thank Paul Dinas for formulating this project. Sonia Weiss had the most difficult job of all—editing and organizing the book into chapters to go along with the DVD; and she did a wonderful job! Lynn Northrup was also instrumental in adding her organizational touch and editing skills. Thanks to Tricia Liebig for her copyediting, and Billy Fields for overseeing the process. Ron Barker and the other excellent photographers—Louis Tallant, Shelli Harrel, and Lisa Brunetti—captured the skill and energy of the beautiful fitness models, Fran Whitehead and Lindsey Brundidge, who made shooting the photos and DVD a lot of fun. Brad Ruekberg went above and beyond by directing, producing, shooting, and editing the DVD.

And once again I must thank my awesome wife Danese and our five children, Alaina, Grant, Laura, Susanna, and Julia, for testing out some of the fitness boxing moves at home before using them in the studio.

Special Thanks to the Technical Reviewer

The Complete Idiot's Guide to Fitness Boxing Illustrated was reviewed by an expert who double-checked the accuracy of what you'll learn here, to help us ensure that this book gives you everything you need to know about fitness boxing. Special thanks are extended to Allen Jackson.

Allen is a Regents Professor of Kinesiology, Health Promotion, and Recreation at the University of North Texas, Denton, Texas. He is a fellow in the American College of Sports Medicine and the American Academy of Kinesiology and Physical Education. He is the author of several books and more than 100 refereed articles in the field of health-related physical fitness. He has maintained a life-long commitment to a healthy lifestyle that includes regular physical activity.

Trademarks

All terms mentioned in this book that are known to be or are suspected of being trademarks or service marks have been appropriately capitalized. Alpha Books and Penguin Group (USA) Inc. cannot attest to the accuracy of this information. Use of a term in this book should not be regarded as affecting the validity of any trademark or service mark.

Century is a registered trademark of Century Incorporated.

In This Part

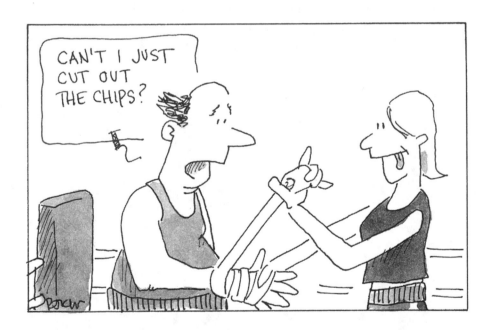

Getting Ready to Rumble

Everybody wants a great body, but where do you start? You might have tried the latest diet or exercise fad and lasted maybe a month. There's so much misinformation about how to get a lean and tight body that you're ready to give up. Don't give up. Fitness boxing might be the last exercise program that you'll ever need.

Part 1 introduces you to what fitness boxing is all about and gives you the foundation to make your commitment to the program. You'll get an introduction to the theories behind the offensive and defensive moves that are at the core of fitness boxing.

In This Chapter

- ◆ What fitness boxing is—and what it isn't
- ◆ How fitness boxing builds great bodies
- ◆ The benefits of fitness boxing
- ◆ A few pointers before you begin
- ◆ Keeping things safe
- ◆ What a typical fitness boxing workout looks like

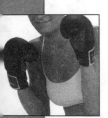 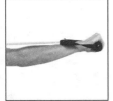 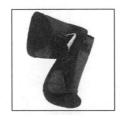 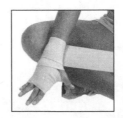 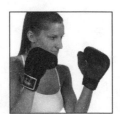 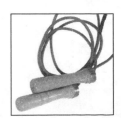

Chapter 1

Why Choose Fitness Boxing?

If someone were to tell you about an exercise program that could firm your shoulders, flatten your abs, chisel your hips, sculpt your legs, and tone your back and arms in just minutes a day, and they told you the program was easy, affordable, and fun, wouldn't you want to jump on that particular bandwagon?

If your answer is yes, fitness boxing is for you.

In this chapter, you learn more about what fitness boxing is, understand how it delivers the kinds of results that it does, and find out why it just might be the perfect exercise program for you.

What Is Fitness Boxing?

Fitness boxing (also known as cardio boxing) is a workout that combines traditional boxing moves and training approaches with modern cardiovascular and muscle-conditioning methods. This combination has extraordinary total body conditioning benefits accessible to everyone who wants the best workout of their lives.

In many respects, fitness boxing is a new take on an ancient activity turned sport. People have been sparring from the beginning of recorded history—historians note that boxing appeared as an Olympic event in the seventh century B.C.E. Back then, the sport was more about avoiding your opponent's fists than it was about hitting. Bouts included hitting, kicking, grappling, head-butting, joint-locking, and even choking, and ended when the contestants grew too weary to continue—or when they died.

Boxing disappeared for a number of centuries after the Romans banned it right before the beginning of the Common Era. It reappeared in England in the late 1600s, and over the next few centuries underwent a number of refinements. Boxers used gloves instead of fighting with their bare hands, and they boxed for a specific number of 3-minute rounds instead of continuing on until someone dropped. Hitting below the belt was prohibited, and wrestling or grappling moves that had previously been a part of the sport, were significantly reduced.

Sweet Science

Boxing is generally thought of as a man's sport, at least until fairly recently, but there have been plenty of female boxers over the centuries. According to the Women's Boxing Archives Network, there are records of fights between women going back to the early 1700s. Unlike men, female boxers were allowed to use their hands, knees, and feet in their bouts. Women's boxing was part of the third Olympic Games, and in the 1920s, boxing was part of the physical training program for young women in Boston.

Sports enthusiasts have long known the benefits of training like a boxer; how the moves and the cardio workouts necessary to create enough stamina to go the distance in the ring built strong, lean bodies and hearts conditioned like racehorses. As such, boxing equipment such as speed bags, jump ropes, and heavy bags have long been common in gyms and fitness centers. Some people have even taken boxing lessons and learned how to spar just to reap the benefits of training like a boxer, not necessarily because they had any interest in fighting.

When aerobics classes became the big thing in the 1970s, instructors often included some basic boxing punches and steps to keep routines fresh for class participants. Over time, some classes began to focus more on boxing moves, and another fitness craze was born. Or perhaps better put, reborn.

Today, fitness boxing is a standard component of class rosters at many exercise facilities as more and more people discover the benefits of this type of physical training. As they do, they're also helping to spread the word about a safe, inexpensive exercise approach that builds strong hearts and great-looking muscles that is easy to learn and fun to do. What's more, fitness boxing appeals to both men and women, which makes it a great couples workout, too.

Sweet Science

Hilary Swank trained like a boxer for only three months to prepare for her Oscar-winning role in the 2004 movie *Million Dollar Baby*. Her buff, toned body is testimony to how effective boxing workouts are.

Unlike contact boxing, in fitness boxing you don't have to worry about protecting various body parts from coming into contact with someone else's fists, which means you'll never come out of a fitness boxing session sporting a shiner. About the only protection you'll need are hand wraps and practice gloves if you decide you want to work out with a heavy bag. But here's what's so great about fitness boxing—you can get a great workout without hitting anything at all. You can if you want to, but it's not a requirement of the program.

What Fitness Boxing Is Not

As previously mentioned, fitness boxing is non-contact boxing. It isn't an exercise or training program designed to prepare you for sparring or ring fighting, although you might decide to do one or the other, or both, at some point along the way.

Also, unlike some other self-defense or martial arts-style exercise programs, such as krav maga, tae kwon do, and karate, fitness boxing itself won't prepare you for defending yourself, because you don't make physical contact with your partner. Although fitness boxing is not a full-blown self-defense program, a great side benefit is that you learn some self-defense moves that will help you move more confidently wherever you are. This added confidence can make you less of a target should you find yourself in a threatening situation.

Fitness boxing also isn't cardio-kicking or kickboxing. Although you'll get a great lower-body workout, it doesn't involve the kicks that these programs call for, which can be difficult to learn correctly and carry a higher potential for injury.

Building Great Bodies

For starters, fitness boxing is simply fun. When you're having fun, you're more likely to stick with any exercise program, which will improve your general level of fitness and keep you healthier in the long run. But with fitness boxing, while you're enjoying yourself you're also benefiting from an exercise approach that conditions the body and burns fat like none other. What's more, it works faster and delivers better results than just about any other fitness program out there. Fitness boxing is so effective because you use your whole body and there is so much

variety that your muscles are always guessing what comes next. Fitness boxing borrows different components of exercise from different disciplines to hone your body fast—and the results will last. You do moves to improve your strength, endurance, flexibility, power, and balance.

How? Improving your health and fitness calls for two things: cardiovascular conditioning and building muscular strength and endurance. Fitness boxing's unique combination of traditional boxing moves and training techniques, coupled with modern cardiovascular and muscle training techniques, can, simply put, get you into the greatest condition of your life.

Greater Intensity = More Calorie Burn

Boxing workouts are intense. So are fitness boxing workouts. A typical fitness boxing workout consists of a series of 3-minute sessions, or rounds (just like in the boxing ring) of intense activity, during which time you never stop moving. You might spend those 3 minutes shadow-boxing while performing the boxer's shuffle. Or you might jump rope or hit the heavy bag. Regardless of what you do, you're going to do it as hard as you can for those 3 minutes, then you get to rest for a minute. Then you begin the next 3-minute session. Fitness boxing is simply a form of interval training, a training method that athletes of many sports, including track and swimming, have used for many years. But fitness boxing is more fun and has a natural variety of activity to keep it interesting.

Simply put, intense activity, even when interspersed with short pauses, burns more calories than longer, lower-intensity workouts do. As an example, if you weigh 155 pounds and you're at an average fitness level, you'll burn approximately 280 calories running at a pace of 5 mph for 30 minutes (add some *wind sprints* to this fairly leisurely run, and you'll burn even more calories). It would take you about an hour to burn the same amount of calories walking 3 mph—about the pace you'd be at if you took your dog for a nice, leisurely walk.

Clear as a Bell

Wind sprints call for moving faster than normal during activity so that you feel "winded." Advanced athletes need to move very fast (sprint) to reach this state; beginners might feel winded when walking fast.

Although the following chart is more for boxing than for fitness boxing, it'll give you an idea of the calorie burn for various boxing workouts for three weight classes. Workout length is one hour.

	130 lbs.	155 lbs.	190 lbs.
General boxing workout	708	844	1,035
Punching bag	354	422	518
Sparring	531	633	776

Source: www.nutristrategy.com/activitylist4.htm

If you're just starting a fitness program, fitness boxing can help you see results faster than many other forms of exercise, which can be a great incentive to sticking with things until you reach your goals. If you're a long-time exerciser and you've reached a plateau in your quest for a firmer, fitter body, adding a couple of fitness boxing sessions a week to your fitness program can serve as the catalyst to break you through

that plateau and help you reach higher fitness levels. Trying to lose a couple of pounds quickly so you'll look great for that high school reunion? Fitness boxing will help get you there faster.

Knockout Punch

Fitness boxing is a fantastic cross-training activity, but depending on what your fitness goals are, you might not want to make it the primary focus of your exercise program. If you're working toward running a marathon or plan to compete in any other type of endurance sport, you'll still want to devote a fair amount of your time to training specifically for those sports, and to building longer workouts in your overall program to prepare your body for them.

Intense workouts are also great stamina builders. As you progress in your fitness boxing program, you'll find that over time, workouts feel easier and you last longer. What's more, the stamina you build doing fitness boxing will give you more energy outside of your workouts as well.

More Muscle = More Calorie Burn

Fitness boxing is similar to other full-body sports, such as cross-country skiing and rowing, in that it engages virtually every muscle group in your body. The more muscles you use, the more calories you burn and the more fat you lose. It's as simple as that.

Taking things a step further, if you increase the amount of muscle on your frame, you'll continue to burn more fat and stay leaner, and fitness boxing is great for doing this, too.

However, unlike other full-body sports, fitness boxing constantly challenges your muscles in new ways because it involves so many different activities. Instead of doing the same exercise the same way over and over again, you mix things up. This builds and tones muscles using two proven muscle-building approaches.

Muscle Confusion

Changing what you do on a regular basis builds muscle by putting them in a state of confusion, otherwise known as—you guessed it—muscle confusion. Because your muscles never quite know what to expect, they don't get bored and they keep on developing and getting firmer.

Muscle confusion also calls for varying the angle of your exercise, and fitness boxing is unparalleled for this. As an example, when you use weight machines, you work your muscles at the same or nearly the same angle all the time. If you do the same exercise the same way all the time, your muscles get used to the same movement. They'll reach a certain point and not develop any farther.

Although walking and jogging are fine and lifting weights in a straight line is okay, most everything you do in your life requires you to move at different angles.

When you challenge your muscles at different angles, you recruit more muscle fibers to do the work, and this stimulates them to grow strong and firm. The more muscle fibers you involve in your activities, the sooner you'll achieve a firm, toned boxer's physique.

The unique combination of moves found in fitness boxing builds definition, not bulk, and develops functional muscle—that is, muscle that helps you do things that take strength, such as changing a tire or hauling groceries around.

Progressive Overload

Fitness boxing also uses the theory of *progressive overload* to build strength and tone muscles.

As an example, you might do a heavy bag routine one day and use resistance bands the next. Each activity calls for throwing punches, and you'll use some muscles to extend your arm and other muscles to pull your arm back. To increase the intensity of the movement—that is, overload the muscle—you can add weight, do more repetitions (reps), or intensify the movement itself; for example, hit the bag harder.

Clear as a Bell

Progressive overload refers to gradually increasing the intensity of a workout. As intensity increases, muscles get overloaded, and overloading muscles is what makes them stronger.

Whether you hit a bag, use exercise bands, dumbbells, or a medicine ball, the goal is to progressively overload your muscles as you move through the exercise to completion. In other words, you intensify the activity in some way to make it progressively harder until you can't do it anymore. Overloading your muscles is what makes them stronger. When you overload your muscles during a fitness boxing workout and take a couple days to recover, your muscles respond by becoming stronger for your next workout. Increased strength also translates into increased muscle tone.

Resistance training, which is an excellent way to build muscle, is also a part of fitness boxing. You can use exercise bands, dumbbells, and medicine balls to train your muscles at a variety of speeds and movements, and get results that you could never accomplish on a bulky weight machine.

More Fitness Boxing Benefits

Here are just a few more reasons why you'll want to make fitness boxing a part of your life:

◆ **Workouts are flexible.** If you don't have time for a full fitness boxing workout, you can split your training into parts. If you like to run, do your roadwork in the morning, bring your jump rope to work for a before-lunch jump-a-thon, and do some boxing drills in the evening.

◆ **It helps the time-crunched.** You can replace traditional weight-training routines with a punching-bag program twice a week and train all your upper-body muscle groups simultaneously in half the time. How? When you land a punch, you not only work the muscles on the side you're throwing the punch from, you also work the muscles on the opposite side of your body, just in a different way. This gives you more bang for your buck because you work more muscle groups in a shorter amount of time.

◆ **It fits anywhere.** You can individualize fitness boxing to meet your needs, and add fitness boxing moves for variety in your existing exercise program. Include a few punches in your running routine or skip rope after you lift weights. You can shadowbox anytime, anywhere. And you don't need any equipment or a partner.

◆ **It's portable.** You can customize your fitness boxing workouts to fit your mood or environment. Choose to hit the bag or practice your footwork on a rainy day. When the weather clears, go outside for some fitness boxing roadwork drills. Fitness boxing can be performed in a hotel room, outdoors, or in your own home.

◆ **It releases excess stress.** Punching a bag is a great way to work out things that get under your skin. As you take out your frustrations on an inanimate object, your brain releases feel-good chemicals called endorphins, helping you move from a distressed mental state to a positive one.

◆ **It cures exercise boredom.** Fitness boxing involves such a variety of activities that you seldom get bored or suffer overuse injuries that are common to repetitive motion activities, such as running. You'll also learn skills you never would on a stepper or treadmill.

◆ **It's easy.** Fitness boxing doesn't require memorizing endless choreography or tricky dance steps.

◆ **It's cheap.** You don't have to spend a dime on equipment if you don't want to. If you do buy equipment, you won't have to spend an arm and a leg to get a great setup. A couple hundred dollars will buy you a bag, gloves, jump rope, timer, and maybe some music.

◆ **It gives you better all-around performance.** If you practice other sports, you'll find that you will have better stamina, increased strength, increased speed, and increased coordination.

Sweet Science

Although boxing appears to be an upper-body activity, your lower body does 75 percent of the work, as it's this part of your body that powers your punches and blocks. As such, your lower body gets extra bonus workout points when you perform fitness boxing balance and footwork drills.

Some Pointers Before You Begin

Fitness boxing is so much fun and so easy to learn that it's easy to get overeager and hit it really hard at first. This is never a good idea, regardless of the exercise program, and it's an especially bad idea here. Doing so increases the chances for injury, and can make you so sore that you might think twice about sticking with the program.

To do fitness boxing right, it's important to take your time and learn how to do the traditional punches, upper-body moves, and footwork correctly. Reading this book and following the accompanying DVD will go a long way in showing you the right way to do your fitness boxing workouts.

After you develop a good understanding of the basic moves and develop some muscle memory by practicing them often, you'll be able to design your own combinations and put them together as pieces of a puzzle to create an effective workout. There is no limit to your creativity with your fitness boxing program.

Fitness boxing exercises are designed on the premise that you're right handed. If you're a lefty, you may choose to use the opposite hand that a right-handed person would use. You would throw a right jab instead of a left jab. Instead of a right cross you would throw a left cross.

You can also choose to do fitness boxing from a right-handed stance. If you play golf right handed or hit right handed, even if you're a lefty, you might prefer this. Many left-handed people feel very comfortable in a right-handed stance.

If you're left handed, and you do decide to use the southpaw stance, then just as you do with the rest of the right-handed world, switch the punches around—right jab, left cross, right hook. That's it. No big deal.

The Usual Cautionary Statement

As mentioned, fitness boxing is an extremely safe form of exercise when done correctly. If you take things slowly and follow the instructions in this book, coupled with the instructions on the accompanying DVD, you'll be well on your way to learning how to do fitness boxing right.

However, before beginning your fitness boxing program, it's a good idea to take some simple precautions. Getting the okay from your personal physician before launching into a new fitness program is always advised and is simply good sense. It's no different with fitness boxing.

If it's been awhile since you've had a complete physical, it's strongly suggested that you get one before you start your fitness boxing program. If you have any concerns about your cardiovascular health, ask for a resting EKG at the very least. An exercise stress test is even better. Fitness boxing is intense. You want to be sure your body is up to the task. This is one thing about which it is very good to be safe rather than sorry.

Also as previously discussed, because fitness boxing is new and exciting, you may be tempted to do too much too soon. Begin slowly and progress gradually. Learning fitness boxing techniques and conditioning is a slow process, and is meant to be learned step by step. Let your learning and your progress take as long as it needs to take. Don't rush things.

Although it might not seem like it now, learning the basic boxing moves, even at a walking pace, is a workout in itself. After you get the moves down, and you speed things up for a 3-minute round of high-intensity punching, you'll develop a new respect for the guys—and gals—who duke it out in the ring, practicing what aficionados call the "sweet science" of boxing.

Inside a Typical Fitness Boxing Training Session

Now that you know a little bit more about what fitness boxing is, you might be curious to know what an actual training session might be like. Although no two sessions are the same, the following is a fairly typical one. This particular workout calls for practicing all the basic punches for 3-minute intervals, and will last for approximately 30 minutes, not including warm up and cool down.

Although there are as many different fitness boxing workouts as there are people doing them, there's one thing that stays consistent—the length of each exercise interval. Three-minute rounds—the same length of time as rounds in a boxing match—are the standard, and are as much as you'll be able to take when you're going all out.

You might not be familiar with all the terminology now, but don't worry about that. You'll learn it as you go through this book and the DVD. Here's what a basic workout might look like:

Warm up: Easy shadowboxing for 3 minutes, followed by 30 seconds of a calf stretch exercise, and 3 minutes of easy jump roping. Total warm up: 6.5 minutes.

Take a 1-minute break while you put on your hand wraps and bag gloves.

Workout: Begin with one 3-minute round divided into the following six 30-second intervals. Set your timer so it buzzes or dings every 30 seconds.

30 seconds—Left jab.

30 seconds—Right cross.

30 seconds—Left hook.

30 seconds—Alternate left and right uppercuts.

30 seconds—Put all punches together and come up with your own creative combinations.

30 seconds—High-intensity round of combinations. Go for the burn and impress the judges!

1-minute break.

Practice all basic punches on the bag for 3 minutes.

1-minute break.

Do a few combinations for 3 minutes. Finish with an all-out 30-second bagwork blitz.

Take a 1-minute break to remove your bag gloves and hand wraps. Prepare for roadwork. Jog one block, run one block, jog one block. Continue jog/run for 10 minutes.

Cool down: Light shadowboxing. Then take a few minutes to stretch it out. Total cool down: 6.5 minutes.

That's it! Looks like fun, doesn't it? Now it's time to get started on the workout of your life!

The Least You Need to Know

◆ Fitness boxing takes traditional boxing moves and training methods and combines them with the latest cardiovascular and muscle-conditioning methods.

◆ Improving your health and fitness requires two things: cardiovascular conditioning and building muscular strength and endurance. Fitness boxing is a stellar approach to doing both.

◆ Fitness boxing moves, like boxing in general, are designed from the right-handed perspective. If you're left handed, you can choose to switch the punches around or learn how to do the moves from a right-handed stance.

◆ Be safe. Get the okay from your personal physician before starting your fitness boxing program.

In This Chapter

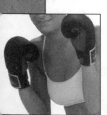
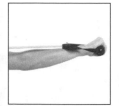
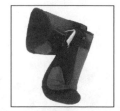
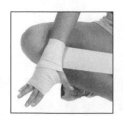
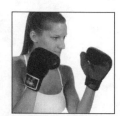
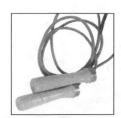

Heating Things Up

The title of this chapter refers to warming up before working out, which is one thing that's definitely not up for debate in the world of exercise and fitness.

Maybe you're so anxious to get going that warming up seems like a waste of time. Maybe you simply don't think it's really necessary. But here's the thing: warming up is not a waste of time, and yes, it's really necessary.

In this chapter, you learn why warming up before you work out is so important. There are also some warm-up routines included that should convert even the biggest diehard.

Warm Muscles = Happy Muscles

Exercise physiologists and others who study the effects of exercise on the human body agree that warming up is a crucial component in exercise. The science behind this is indisputable—warm bodies simply move better than cold ones do. The science behind this gets a little technical, but it's worth getting to know, especially if you're not good about warming up now. If anything's going to convert you, this stuff should.

It's common knowledge that activity boosts the bloodflow to your muscles, and you may know that oxygenated muscles are more pliable and less likely to get injured.

But even more important, increased bloodflow helps eliminate exercise-induced waste products—in particular, lactic acid—from working muscles. Lactic acid is what makes muscles burn, and the discomfort is what makes people want to quit exercising before they're truly tired. Minimizing lactic acid results in longer and more productive workouts.

Even when you don't warm up first, the increased bloodflow during your exercise program will remove some of these waste products. However, when you don't ease into exercise, you're starting at a deficit, and your body has to work harder to do it. It's kind of like starting an engine on a cold morning. You can drive off right away and your car will run okay, but it will run better if you give it a minute or two to warm up.

Sweet Science

In a recent study of 12 women published in *Medicine & Science in Sports & Exercise*, researchers reported that warming up before exercise resulted in significantly less lactic acid buildup. The results came from studies conducted on 12 women; six actively warmed up before exercise, the others did not.

It's not the worst thing in the world if you skip a warm up every so often, or if you warm up for less time than you should occasionally. However, the effects of not warming up are somewhat cumulative, so it's a good idea not to skip this step very often. Your muscles won't be as effective at removing waste products as they could be, and your workouts won't be as efficient as they could be. Plus, you'll be at an increased risk for injuries.

If you don't have a lot of time to exercise, why would you want to waste it by exercising less efficiently than you could? If you have to make a choice between warming up and working out, warming up is definitely the better choice.

In fitness boxing, warming up provides another important benefit in that it helps you mentally prepare for the intensity of fitness boxing workouts. You get pumped up and your attention gets properly focused.

A good warm up also improves the nerve connections between your brain and your muscles. Muscle contractions speed up, which makes your moves more efficient.

Warm Up How To's

A typical warm up involves a combination of light exercises that gradually increase until you reach a specific intensity.

There are lots of different ways to warm up. You can jog, ride a stationary bike—anything that gets your heart rate up and your blood flowing will work. That said, experts recommend matching your warm up to your workout for maximum effectiveness. So, for example, if you're doing a heavy bag session, you'll want to choose a warm up that primarily focuses on the muscles and moves that you'll use during that workout.

In fitness boxing, however, your warm up can be directly related to boxing moves or simply based on more general moves. Again, anything that gets your heart pumping and increases your body temperature (it comes up naturally as your body works harder) will work.

Corner Man

Having a higher body temperature adds to the benefit of your entire workout. It accelerates the rate of all your bodily processes, speeds up your metabolism, and improves your fat burning.

Regardless of the type of warm up you do, keeping the following points in mind will make it a good one:

◆ Don't rush through your warm up; evaluate how your muscles feel. If you feel any discomfort on any exercise, modify it or skip it all together.

◆ Warm up before you stretch. Never stretch a cold muscle. Your warm-up prepares you for your activity and prevents injury. Stretching a cold muscle may cause injury. Similar to taking a piece of steak out of the freezer; if you try to bend it, it breaks.

◆ Warm up longer on cold days. On warm days, you may be surprised how quickly your body will be ready for action. On cool days it may take twice as long for you to be ready to rumble.

Knockout Punch

The purpose of your warm-up is to get your body temperature up. Don't confuse your warm up with stretching. Be sure that you are actively moving during your warm up.

Because your warm-up only needs to last about five minutes, you can do a variety of warm-up exercises or just do one exercise for the entire five minutes.

A fun warm-up that includes a lot of variety begins with Arm Circles forward for 30 seconds and backward for 30 seconds to loosen up your shoulders. Next, do Boxer's Bends for another minute to warm up your waist. Minute three might include March/Side March/Back March to heat up your hips and lower body. Now you're breaking a sweat so you're ready for Jogging in Place for 1 minute. For your final minute, practice your Boxer's Shuffle. Now you're ready to train. (All the specific moves in this warm-up regimen can be found in the photo section that follows.)

Arm Circles

Arm Circles prepare your shoulders for punching. You should always be able to see your hands with your peripheral vision.

Arm Circles consist of holding arms straight out from your sides. Begin by moving your arms in a small circular motion. As your arms begin to tire, move them in larger circular motions. Then alternate directions.

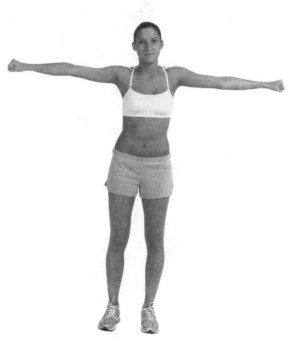

Keep your chest out, stomach in, and back straight. Imagine that the strength to perform Arm Circles is coming from your abdomen.

Joint Circles

Joint Circles are good for checking joint mobility. Because these exercises should be pain free, they're good for taking an inventory of how your body feels. Boxers traditionally perform joint rotation exercises before they train.

Turn each body part clockwise and then counter-clockwise, beginning with your fingers, then your wrists, elbows, shoulders, neck, waist, hips, legs, knees, ankles, and toes. Perform slow circular movements until your joints move smoothly.

Practice Joint Circles often until you can do them without thinking. Include them as part of your mental preparation before your workout. As you rotate each joint, imagine what you will be doing during your fitness boxing program.

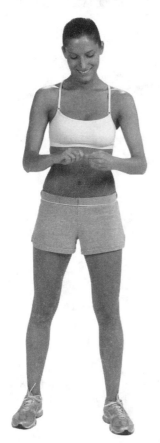

Perform Joint Circles as an inventory of how your body is feeling.

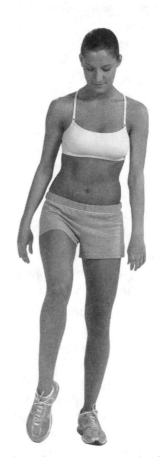

Perform these movements slowly.

Boxer's Bend

Boxer's Bends is an excellent warm-up for the torso. It's also good preparation for the slip, bob, and weave moves of fitness boxing.

With your hands in a fighting position and your knees bent, alternate bending at the waist in four directions. Be sure to keep your back straight and head up. Make small, subtle movements at first. As you get in better shape, make

the moves more pronounced and at a larger range of motion.

Corner Man

Use it or lose it is a truism for Boxer's Bends. Train your body to continue to move in all directions and it will. If you forget to move in one direction, your body won't want to take you there anymore.

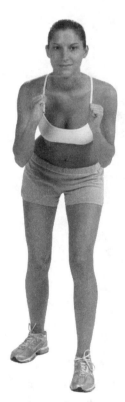
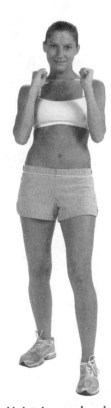
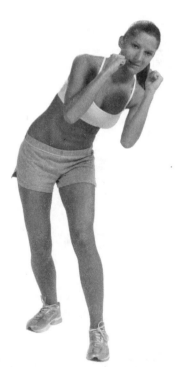
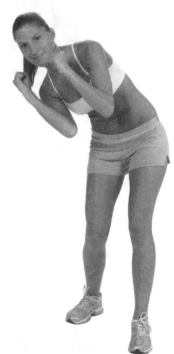

With your hands in the fighting position, lean forward from your waist until you reach a 45-degree angle.

Maintain your hands in the fighting position and lean backward from your waist extending your spine until you feel a light stretch in your abdominals.

While your hands remain in a fighting position, lean slowly to the left a few inches and hold the stretch.

Your final torso stretch is leaning to the right a few inches until you feel the stretch.

March/Side March/ Back March

Marching warms up your lower body. Using your large muscle groups also sparks your fat-burning metabolic furnace.

March in place, side to side, then front and back. Keep your hands up in a fighting position. March forward, then back, then to your right, and then to your left. Control your steps and don't "pound the ground."

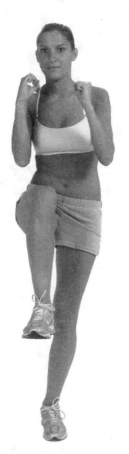

With your hands in a fighting position, march front and back and then side to side in any pattern you desire.

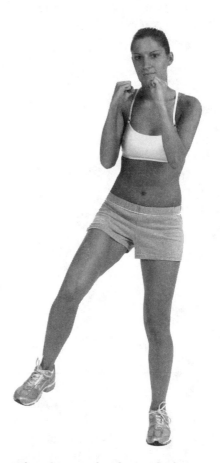

When you march side to side, be sure to move the outside leg first just as you do during your footwork drills.

Cross-Over March

This exercise should feel good as it warms up and stretches out your hips. If you move very slowly during this exercise, your upper legs and buns will get a nice stretch.

Take big cross-over steps to warm up your hips. Cross your right leg over your left and then your left leg over your right.

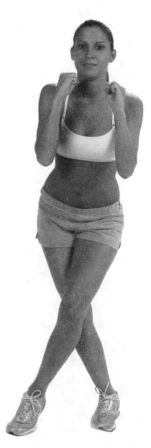

Keep your hands up in a fighting position. Your back should remain straight through the entire exercise. Move as slow as needed to maintain your balance. There is no need to move fast during this exercise.

Knee Lift

This exercise serves as a dynamic warm up and stretch for your buns and hamstrings.

Bring your hands up to chest level with your palms facing downward. Bring each knee up and try to touch your palms with your knees. Move your lower body only; focus on your hip flexors and thighs, which should do all the work. Don't bring your palms down to meet your knees.

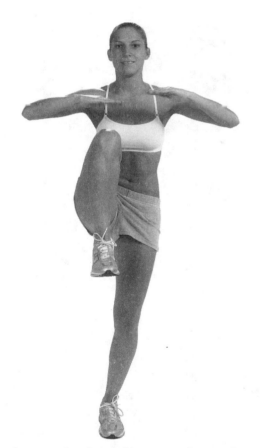

Keep your hands up, chest up, and stomach in. Move your lower body only. Resist the temptation to bring your hands down toward your knees.

Side Twist

Side Twists prepare the upper body for rotation punches such as the hook and cross. This is also a good exercise to do after you've been sitting at your computer for long periods.

Keep your hands in the fighting position and spread your feet shoulder-width apart. Keep your knees slightly bent.

Exhale on each side to side movement. Move slowly and purposefully.

Jog in Place

Keep your hands up in a fighting position and Jog in Place. Don't raise your knees high or kick your heels back toward your hips. Instead, both your knee lift and heel kick should be small movements. Remember, don't "pound the ground."

Corner Man

You usually swing your arms back and forth when you jog. Holding your arms in the fighting position makes this warm-up move a little more difficult, but discipline yourself to keep your arms in this position.

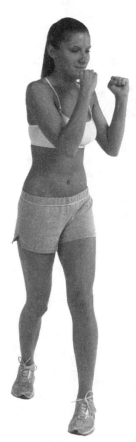
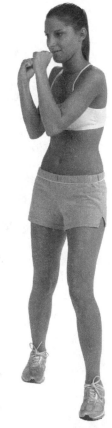

Twist your upper body slowly to the left until you feel a stretch in your waist.

Twist your upper body slowly to the right until you feel a stretch in your waist.

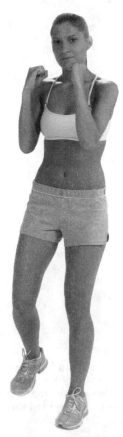

Jog with your chest out and back straight. Breathe from your diaphragm.

Boxer's Shuffle

The Boxer's Shuffle is a must-learn movement pattern. Start by standing sideways to your imaginary opponent with your hands up in the fighting position. Keep your feet shoulder-width apart and step forward with your left foot. Your right foot should slide up and replace the position of your left foot.

As your lead foot steps, the other foot follows immediately as if there were a two foot rope tied to your ankles. Keep both knees bent when you shuffle so that your head doesn't bob up and down. Keep your upper body relaxed and exhale through pursed lips on each shuffle.

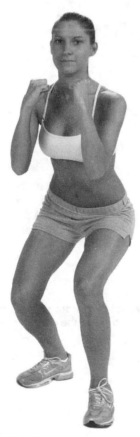

Maintain a relaxed posture and stay on the balls of your feet.

Half Jump (No Impact) with Support

This exercise is a great warm-up for your lower body. Because it doesn't require foot to floor impact, it's also easy on your joints.

Hold on to a chair and bend your knees at a 45-degree angle. As you extend your knees, do everything you normally would do if you were going to jump, but keep your feet on the floor.

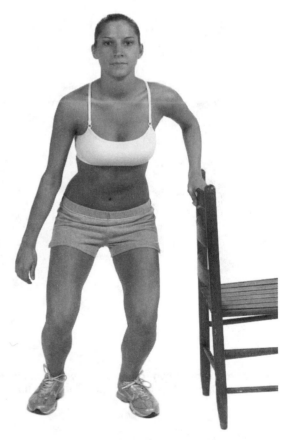

Keep your chest out and stomach in. Hold on to the chair lightly to help you keep your balance. When you extend your knees, just before full extension, decelerate so your feet do not leave the floor.

Full Jump (No Impact) with Support

This exercise is a great warm up for your lower body. Like the previous move, it doesn't require foot to floor impact.

Hold on to a chair and bend your knees at a 90-degree angle. As you extend your knees, do everything you normally would do if you were going to jump, without leaving the floor.

If your knees bother you when you bend at a 90-degree angle, stick with the Half Jump with Support exercise.

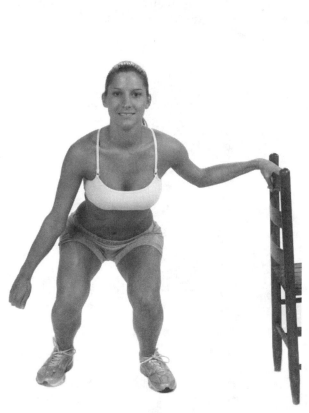

Be sure to maintain correct posture as you drop into a squat position with your thighs parallel to the floor.

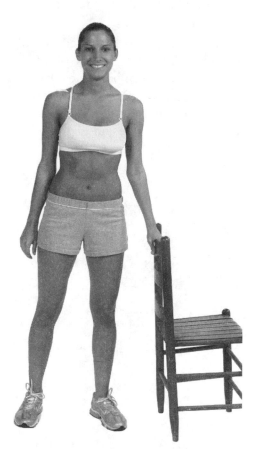

Extend your knees from your squat position and hold on to the chair for balance.

Half Jump (No Impact)

This exercise is essentially the same as doing Half Squats except that instead of moving 3 seconds in each direction, on the upward motion you accelerate as if you were going to jump.

Just before you extend your knees, decelerate so that your feet do not leave the floor.

With your hands up in the fighting position, perform a Half Jump without having your feet leave the floor.

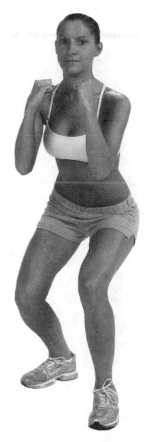

Bend your knees slowly until you reach a 45-degree angle.

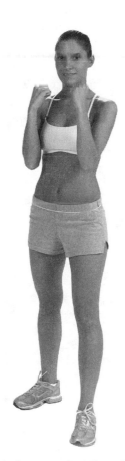

Explode upward until just before your knees are fully extended.

Full Jump with Support

This exercise is a dynamic power drill that warms you up and burns a lot of calories. If you have any orthopedic injuries in your feet, shins, knees, hips, or back, keep your feet on the ground for this exercise.

With your right hand in the fighting position and your left hand holding a chair, perform a Full Jump. When you extend your knees and your feet leave the floor, prepare to land softly with your knees bent, on the balls of your feet and then your heels.

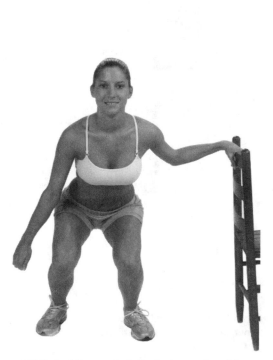

While holding a chair for balance, bend from your knees and prepare to jump.

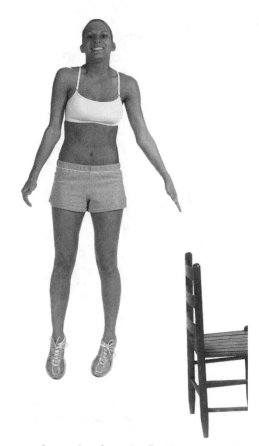

Jump a few inches from the floor. Do not attempt to jump too high.

Skipping

Skipping is a great way to establish a rhythm that you can take with you into your fitness boxing drills.

Keep your hands up in a fighting position and Skip in place at a rhythm of your choice. Stay light on your feet and relaxed throughout the exercise.

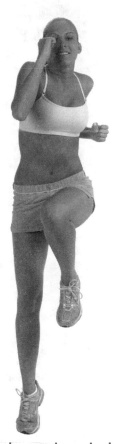

Keep your hands up and your back straight.

 # Power Skipping

Power Skipping warms you up, burns a ton of calories, and is a great power drill.

Power Skipping is the same as Skipping except that you raise your knees higher with each repetition. Propel your knees as high as possible with each repetition. Land on the balls of your feet as softly as you can between each repetition

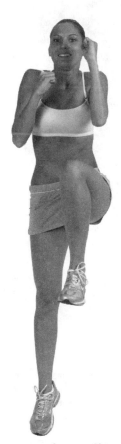

Use your knees to propel yourself in the air. Keep your hands in a fighting stance throughout the exercise.

Jumping Jack Punch

Jumping Jack Punch is similar to jumping jacks, but instead of clapping your hands overhead, you throw punches to the front.

Move your feet from shoulder-width apart and bring them together. When your feet move to shoulder-width apart, throw simultaneous punches with both arms to the front.

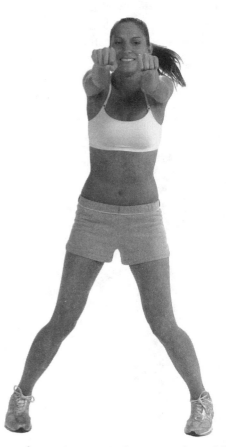

Perform a jumping jack move and straddle your feet while you simultaneously punch with both arms to the front.

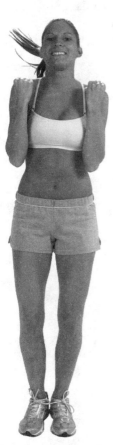

When you bring your feet together, retract your arms to your sides.

Half Squat

Bend your knees until your thighs are at a 45-degree angle to the floor. Keep your hands in a fighting stance throughout your entire set of repetitions. Don't bend your knees too much. This is bad for your knee ligaments.

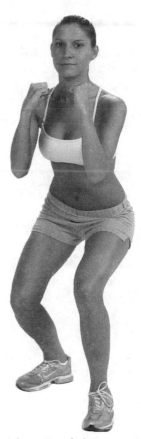

Keep your hands up in a fighting position and bend your knees at a 45-degree angle. Return to your original position keeping your back straight and head up.

Quick Feet

This exercise warms you up and improves your ability to move your feet very quickly.

Take small steps alternating your feet as quickly as you can while pumping your arms vigorously to increase your speed. Move a few feet forward and then a few feet backward.

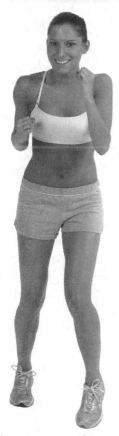

Stand in a fighting stance with correct form. Keep your arms up and move your feet as quickly as you can. Use your arms in a pumping action to move faster.

Warming Up with a Jump Rope

Jumping Rope improves your balance, posture, reflexes, speed, balance, coordination, and reaction time. It tones your forearms, shoulders, abs, and calves. Jumping Rope for 10 minutes at a moderate pace is the rough equivalent to running one mile in 12 minutes.

Start off Jump Roping in one spot. Begin by alternating 15 seconds of jumping with 15 seconds of turning the rope alongside your body without jumping. Over time, do less rope turns and more jumping. Your goal is to jump continuously for 10 minutes. As you begin to improve, increase your speed for 15 seconds of every minute, and begin to move forward and backward. Then as you get more comfortable, begin to move side to side, and then move in a circular pattern.

Keep your shoulders relaxed and your elbows in close to your body just as you do during your fitness boxing drills. Jump just high enough to barely clear the rope. Keep your hands close to your body and use your wrists to turn the rope. Your feet leave the floor only once between each turn of the rope.

Jumping can be hard on the feet, so be sure to wear a good pair of cross-training shoes. Avoid hard surfaces. Jump on wooden floors, cushioned carpet, or rubber tiles.

Corner Man

Doing the same two-foot bounce over and over can feel like torture. Change your jumping style every 15 seconds or so. Move from a Single Jump to a Knee Up, then to a Skip, then a Double Jump, and finally a Boxer's Shuffle.

How to Jump

Grab a handle in each hand and hold each end of the rope at hip level. Let the rope touch the back of your heels. Look straight ahead with your elbows close to your body, forearms down and out at 45-degree angles. Your hands should be about 8 inches from your hips and your thumbs out as if you were hitchhiking with both hands.

Begin turning the rope by making small circles with your wrists. Keep your upper arms almost stationary—your wrists, not your arms, are what power the rope. Keep your elbows bent and hold your arms out to your sides at about hip level. Spin the rope quickly and, as it approaches your toes, skip over it. Jump less than an inch, just high enough to clear the rope. The rope should lightly skim the floor.

Your legs act as shock absorbers and springs that push you off the floor. Stay low, and bend your knees slightly to help absorb the impact. Land softly on the balls of your feet. Your heels should never touch the floor. If possible, use a mirror to check your form.

You might only get five jumps in a row without missing. Ten consecutive jumps is excellent for your first workout. For the first week, concentrate on coordination. Later you can think about cardio.

Rope Turns with Knee Bend

This is a good way to ease into jumping. Turn the rope from your wrist and bend your knees at a 35-degree angle on each rotation of the rope.

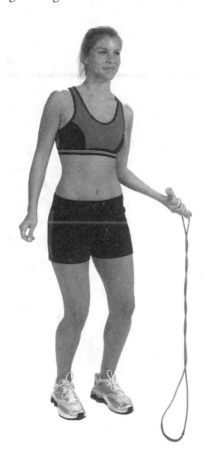

Maintain correct posture throughout this exercise. If your arm begins to fatigue, switch arms and continue.

Knockout Punch

Your calf muscles take quite a beating from jumping rope and fitness boxing drills. Be sure to do Toe Raises to strengthen the shin muscles and do Calf Stretches to balance the strength and flexibility of your lower leg muscles.

 ## Rope Turns with Toe Raise

This exercise strengthens your shin muscles to balance your calves. Do Rope Turns with Toe Raises instead of jumping. Raise your toes off the floor with each revolution of the rope. Balance on your heels.

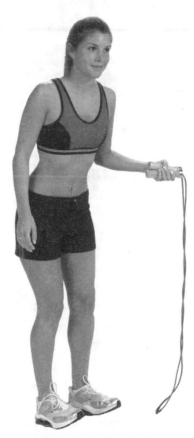

Turn the rope with your wrists. Raise your toes off the floor balancing on the edge of your heels. Maintain correct posture as you keep your weight on your heels.

Propeller Swing (No Jump)

Grab both handles in your left hand and snap the rope to your left side like a whip. Then cross-over to your right side and back again like a propeller. Switch hands and repeat. This is a fantastic upper body exercise that takes your arms and shoulders through a full range of motions.

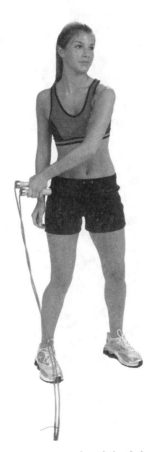

Stand with correct posture and with both handles of the rope in your left hand.

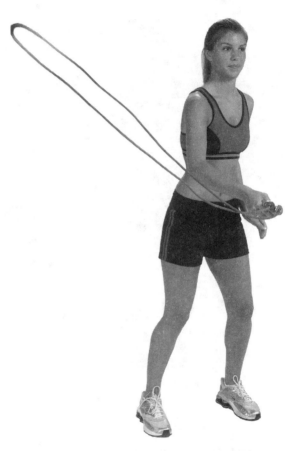

Swing the rope back and forth across your body as quickly as you can while maintaining a flat back.

Figure 8

Grab the handles in both hands and repeat this Figure 8 pattern across your entire body.

Sweep the rope across your entire body using both hands to turn the rope.

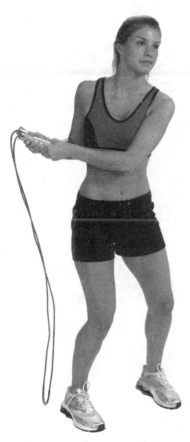

Keep your head up, chest out, and back straight while holding both handles of your rope in both hands.

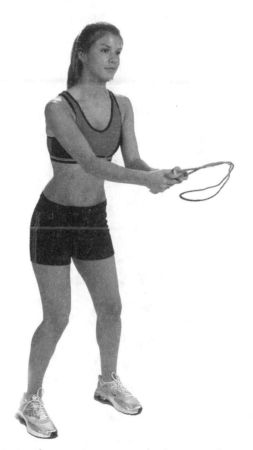

Swing the rope across your body using all your torso muscles to stabilize the movement.

Double Jump

This is a relaxing way to ease into jumping, as it's slower and less demanding than Single Jumps. Simply take two jumps per swing of the rope. Remember to use your wrists to turn the rope. Keep your elbows in and your head up.

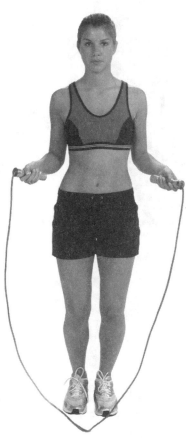

Keep your upper body relaxed and turn the rope with your wrists.

 ## Forward and Back

Begin in a Boxer's Crouch. Hold your elbows in close to your body. Jump an inch forward and an inch back with each revolution of the rope.

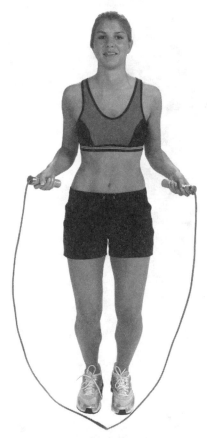

Keep your upper body relaxed and your eyes forward. Hop forward a couple inches on a revolution of the rope and then hop back on the next swing. Continue this forward and back movement through the duration of the routine.

Skier

This move is similar to a skier's slalom motion. Keep your feet together, then jump an inch to the left and an inch to the right. You can do this as a Double Jump if a Single Jump is too difficult.

 Corner Man

Although rope jumping appears to train just your calf muscles, you are actually training your whole body. You must hold your abs and your shoulders back, which trains your entire core.

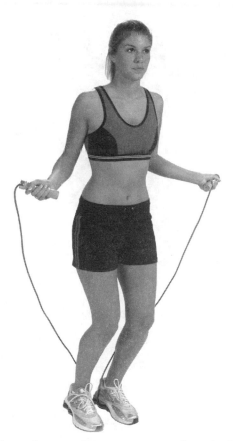

Bend your knees to keep your center of gravity low.

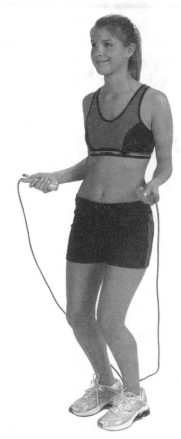

Turn the rope with your wrists and jump very low to the floor.

Straddle

After the rope has cleared your feet, jump into a Side Straddle Hop opening your feet to shoulder width, like the bottom of a jumping jack. Bring legs together on the next revolution. Continue this cycle for the duration of your routine.

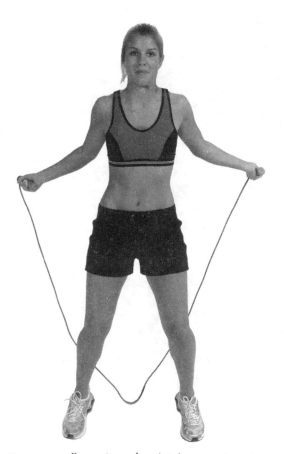

Keep your elbows in and maintain correct posture.

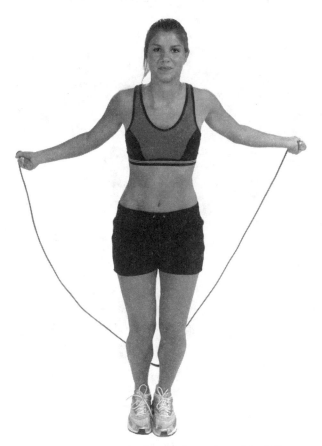

Keep your upper body still throughout this drill.

Jog in Place

Alternate feet as if you're Jogging in Place. Maintain correct posture as you kick your heel toward your hip on each jogging step.

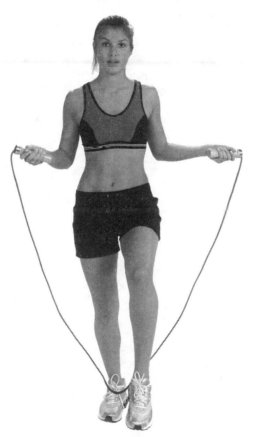

Jog easy with correct posture on the balls of your feet.

High March

This is the same as Jogging in Place except that you bring the knees high. Lift your knees only a few inches at first. Add an inch a week until you are lifting your knees so that your thigh is parallel to the floor on each repetition.

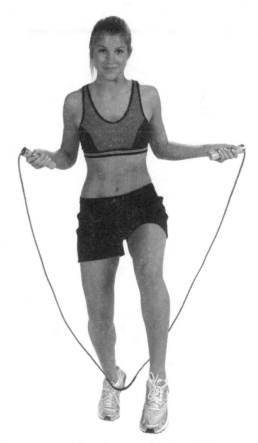

Concentrate on keeping your back straight as you may have a tendency to hunch forward to get your knee up.

Jump Rope Shuffle

This move will make you feel like a real boxer. Start jumping. As the rope approaches your toes, shift your weight slightly to the left and move your left foot a couple of inches forward as you jump. Stay low and bend your knees.

On the next revolution, shift your weight to your right foot and do the same thing. Continue shifting your weight back and forth and scissoring your feet forward and back as you jump.

Bounce once or twice on each leg, depending on how you feel.

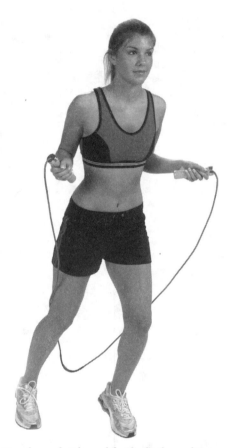

Develop a back-and-forth rhythm when you perform this routine. Resist the temptation to watch your feet.

The Least You Need to Know

- Warming up is very important to prevent injury. It lubricates your joints, increases the temperature in your muscles, and prepares your body for action.

- If you don't think you have time to warm up, you're the type of person who needs to warm up the most.

- Don't rush through your warm-up; evaluate how your muscles feel. If you feel any discomfort on any exercise, modify it or skip it all together.

- Warm up before you stretch. Never stretch a cold muscle. Your warm-up prepares you for your activity and prevents injury.

- Warm up longer on cold days. On warm days, you may be surprised how quickly your body will be ready for action. On cool days it may take twice as long for you to be ready to rumble.

- Start slow when doing Jump Rope drills. Begin by alternating 15 seconds of jumping with 15 seconds of turning the rope alongside your body without jumping. Over time, do fewer rope turns and more jumping.

In This Chapter

- ◆ Keeping your legs strong
- ◆ The basics of leg workouts
- ◆ Moves for shape and definition
- ◆ The king of the lower body moves

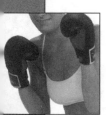
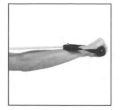
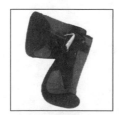
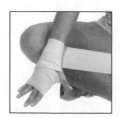
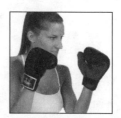
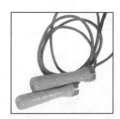

Chapter 3

Stepping It Up

As your legs move, so moves your body. In boxing as well as other sports, your legs are the first part of your body to fatigue, so you must keep them strong.

Well-defined legs, firm glutes, and toned calves can be yours if you do the moves in this chapter.

All About the Legs

Because your lower body muscles are larger than your upper body muscles, leg workouts are great calorie burners. But their benefits go way beyond this. Your legs power your punch.

That said, lots of people don't like leg workouts for one main reason: They're hard! When you train large muscle groups such as your thighs, hamstrings, and buns, it feels like work.

Training your legs with the fitness boxing weight program will also improve the tone in your upper body, as both your upper and lower body muscles work to stabilize your movement.

Leg Workout Basics

Because it's so challenging, lower body training requires extra motivation. It's a good idea to mentally prepare for leg day before you begin your workout. Take a few minutes to close your eyes and imagine what your legs will look like after a few months of training—toned, well-shaped, and defined. Now visualize yourself moving through a few of the fitness boxing leg exercises. "Feel" a sense of energy and power as you mentally rehearse several of the exercises. Open your eyes and begin your warm-up.

When you start your workout, ease into it. Choose resistance that you can comfortably control. Start with some easy repetitions, and then gradually increase the intensity.

You might find yourself holding your breath when you're working your legs due to the exertion level of these exercises. Try not to do this. Always breathe normally during any exercise. Time your exhalations during muscle contractions, and inhale on the short rest between each contraction.

Maintaining good posture is important. Keep your stomach in, relax your neck, and keep your back flat (don't arch). Focus your concentration on the specific muscle group that you're training. Completely contract the muscle you're working on every repetition.

Don't bend your knees so far that they travel beyond your toes. Doing so puts you at risk for developing patellar tendonitis, which is inflammation of the tendons around the knee.

Go down only as far as your body will allow. At first, this might not be very much. As you gain in strength, you'll be able to go deeper and intensify the moves.

Press through your heels—in other words, don't place most of your weight on the balls of your feet. Instead, focus on keeping your weight back toward your heels. Doing so will target your buns and hamstrings.

Picking the Right Weight and Reps

Because the lower body muscles are so large, they can handle quite a bit of weight. Be sure you're lifting enough—you want to feel these exercises when you're done.

If you're relatively new to exercising in general, just lifting your own body weight might be enough for you. If you're a more experienced exerciser, and you're in good shape, you'll need to add some resistance to boost the effectiveness of these moves.

In the beginning, start with weights that are light enough so you can complete 10 repetitions with perfect form and without straining. As you gain in strength, work toward doing these moves with weights that are approximately 60 to 80 percent of the maximum amount that you can lift for one repetition. As an example, if you can squat 100 pounds for one rep, you'd use two 30-pound dumbbells (60 pounds total) or two 40-pound dumbbells (80 pounds total).

For leg work, a repetition range of between 8 and 12 is ideal. For example, some of the exercises will be so easy that you can accomplish 12 reps, no sweat. Other moves may be so challenging that even without any additional resistance, you can barely complete eight reps.

Sample Lower Body Training Routine

For each lower body training session, pick four exercises from the ones that follow. Do one set of each with a minute's rest between sets.

A sample routine might look like this:

> Boxer's Front Lunge—10 reps
>
> Hip Lift—10 reps
>
> Calf Raise—10 reps
>
> Boxer's Leg Press—10 reps

If you're huffing and puffing between sets, take your time before you attempt the next one. It's better to concentrate on maintaining perfect form than to rush through your workout.

Boxer's Front Lunge

The Boxer's Front Lunge targets your buns, thighs, and hamstrings. It also trains the muscles on the outside and inside of the hips, which work to stabilize the movements.

Hold a pair of light dumbbells in your hands with your arms by your sides. Take a slightly greater (one-foot length) than normal step forward. Plant your lead foot and lower your body straight down until the trailing knee is just above the floor. Keep your torso upright, back flat, and knee in line with your foot. Return to the upright position by pushing off the lead leg to recruit your thigh and hip muscles. Switch legs and repeat.

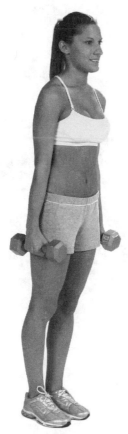

Keep your arms close to your body so that your arms won't tire out before your legs do.

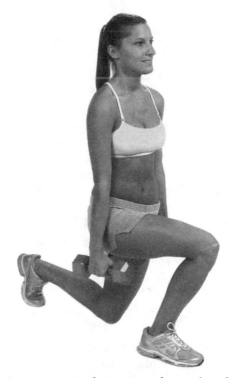

A common mistake is to step forward as if on a tightrope. Instead, keep your feet at least shoulder-width apart.

Boxer's Back Lunge

The Boxer's Back Lunge firms and tones all aspects of your upper leg and is less stressful on your knees.

Hold a pair of light dumbbells in your hands and get into fighting position. Now instead of stepping forward, as you typically would do from this position, take a small step backward with one leg. After a few practice sessions, you can step as far as you would normally step for a basic front lunge. Rest only the ball of that foot on the ground. Your front leg is the working leg.

Now simply lower the knee of your back leg toward the floor. Use your front leg to support your body weight. Perform 10 reps, and then return to the starting position, using your thigh and hip muscles to bring your rear leg back in line with your front leg. Reverse legs, and repeat the exercise again for 10 reps.

Corner Man

If your lightest pair of dumbbells feels too heavy, begin with your hands in the fighting position using only your bag gloves or no weight at all. When you first begin to work out, your body weight is plenty of resistance to receive a training effect.

If you press through your heel, you recruit even more muscle fibers from your buns and hamstrings to firm and tone those hard-to-get, back-of-your-leg muscles. If you prefer to focus on the muscles in the front of your thigh, keep your body weight over the ball of your front foot. And if you want to activate both the front and back of your leg muscles equally, center your weight over the middle of your foot.

Knockout Punch

When you train your legs, protect your lower back at all times by maintaining a neutral spine. That simply means to bend at your hip instead of bending your lower back on any leg exercise.

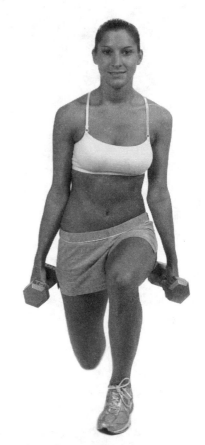

Only descend to the point where you are pain-free. Don't try to go down too far.

Boxer's Angle Lunge

The Boxer's Angle Lunge is extremely effective at building speed and tone as it never gives your muscles a chance to adapt. Changing up angles keeps your muscles guessing.

Hold a pair of light dumbbells in your hands in the fighting position. Your knees should be in line with your toes. Step off to a 45-degree angle keeping your hips square and your back straight. Plant your lead foot and lower your body straight down until the trailing knee is just above the floor. Keep your torso upright and back flat. Return to the upright position by pushing off the lead leg. Perform 10 repetitions with each leg.

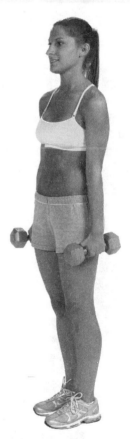

Begin in an upright position with your chest out, stomach in, and elbows in close to your body with the weights in your hands.

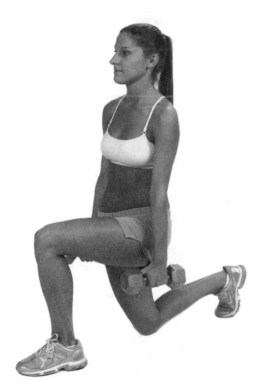

Step off to a 45-degree angle keeping your hips square and your back straight.

Boxer's Lateral Lunge

The Boxer's Lateral Lunge is an excellent inner and outer thigh toner.

Hold a pair of light dumbbells in your hands in the fighting position. Perform a combination of the squat and the lunge by stepping sideways. Plant the lead foot with your toes sideways and squat. Keep the knee pointed over your toes. Push off the lead foot to the start position. Keep your torso upright and back flat. Perform 10 repetitions with each leg. Maintain perfect form on each repetition.

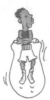

Sweet Science

Performing leg exercises at different angles recruits more muscle fibers so your thighs, hamstrings, and hips will firm and tone at an accelerated pace.

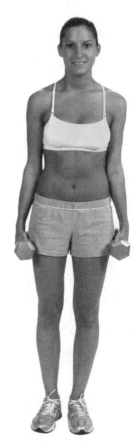

Don't try to step too far sideways with the lead leg. You should feel comfortable as if performing a basic squat.

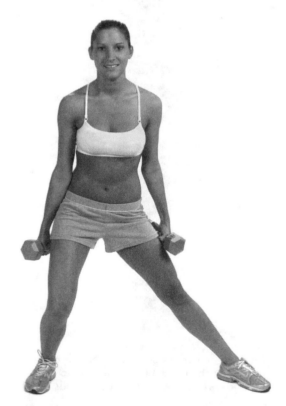

Bend your lead leg into a comfortable position. It's not necessary to bend it at a 90-degree angle.

Bob and Weave Slide

The Bob and Weave Slide is a fat burner and a full-body toning exercise. Your legs start the action and your upper body finishes it.

This exercise is as physically demanding as heavy squats in the weight room. If you begin to feel breathless doing it, slow down. Perform just a few reps each workout until your body adapts.

Stand facing forward with your feet spread a few inches beyond shoulder width. Lean to your left and shift your weight into your left leg. Crouch and slide your right foot in toward

your left foot so that the inside part of your feet almost touch. Bend your left knee so that it supports your body weight on the outside edge of your left foot. Push sideways to the right like a boxer evading a punch, using the power from your left leg to propel you. Slide your right foot, leg, torso, arms, and body to the right like a boxer in motion. As you now lean fully into your right leg, slide your left foot in toward your right leg so that the inside part of your feet almost meet.

Continue this cycle for 10 repetitions. Keep your arms up in fighting position. Focus on shifting your weight smoothly from leg to leg.

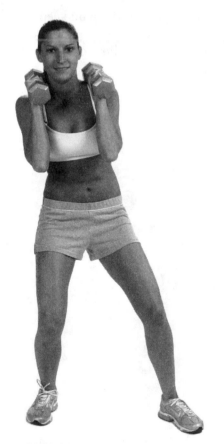

Make small, subtle bob and weave movements until you're comfortable with this exercise.

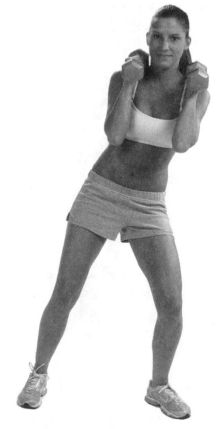

Be sure to keep your back straight. Don't let the weight from the dumbbells pull you forward.

Hip Lift

There is no better exercise to target your buns and hamstrings than the Hip Lift, as this exercise specifically isolates these muscle groups. Other leg exercises such as squats and lunges require you to use your thighs. If your thighs fatigue before the muscles on the back of your legs, then you have to quit. If you quit before your buns and hamstrings are fully activated, then these muscles won't get fully targeted. The Hip Lift requires you to give your full attention to shaping your buns and hamstrings.

Here's how to do it:

1. Stand with a dumbbell in each hand and your arms extended down in front of your body. Keep your elbows and knees soft to protect your joints.

Clear as a Bell _____

Keeping your joints **soft** means keeping them slightly bent. This prevents injury by placing the stress on your muscles instead of your joints.

Keep your back straight as you hinge from the hip and lean forward as the weights are lowered.

When you feel a stretch in you hamstrings and hips, return to your starting position. Be sure to keep your weight in your heels and place your mind into your muscle on each rep.

It's very important that you keep your back straight so that your buns and hamstrings are doing the work instead of your lower back.

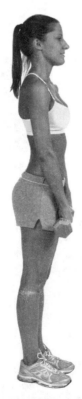

Begin with your chest out, stomach in, and back straight. Keep your elbows and knees soft.

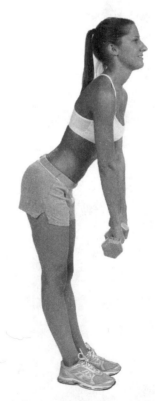

Keep your weight centered over your heels. As soon as you feel the stretch in your hamstrings and hips, slowly return to your starting position for 10 repetitions.

Calf Raise

If you want cut, defined, shapely calves, do Calf Raises.

Stand with a dumbbell in each hand and your arms extended to your sides. Press through the balls of your feet as you raise your heels off the floor. Return to your starting position and continue for 10 repetitions.

Keep your toes straight ahead as it's a fallacy to change your toe position to work different aspects of your calves. Changing the angles of your toes only internally or externally rotates your hips. It has nothing to do with the activation of the muscle fibers in your lower legs.

 ### Corner Man

When you do Calf Raises, start with your heels on the same level as your toes. Although bodybuilders try to achieve that extra stretch in the calf muscle by dropping their heels below their toes on this move, doing so risks injury to the Achilles tendon.

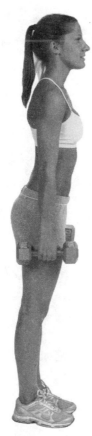

When your heels reach the highest position, hold for a second before returning them to the floor.

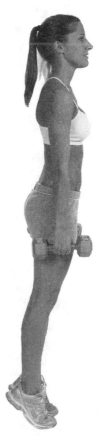

Instead of bouncing through your reps, pay attention to the quality of your movement.

Balance Squat

Balance Squats are a must for firm, shapely thighs and buns. The reason they're so effective is because they concentrate most of the effort on one leg. Focusing on one leg at a time not only allows you to increase the intensity, it also challenges your balancing muscles.

Balance on your right leg with your left leg behind you. Keep your arms up in the fighting position with a dumbbell in each hand. Your elbows are in, hands up, and chin down. Squat with your right leg down to a 45-degree angle. Rise up until the knee is bent slightly. Move 3 seconds down and 3 seconds up for 10 repetitions. Switch legs and repeat.

Although you may be able to squat 150 pounds in the gym, a balance squat is quite a challenge. Not only do you need strength to perform a balance squat, you need coordination, balance, and flexibility to complete the movement.

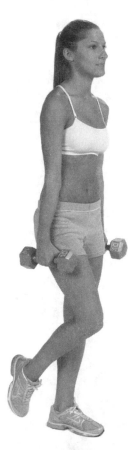

Bend your knee just a few inches until you feel your thighs and hips flex.

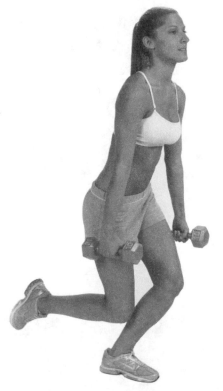

Press through your heels on both the up and down phase of the Balance Squat.

Boxer's Squat

The Boxer's Squat firms and tones both your upper and lower body. Your arms are forced to isometrically contract as they hold the dumbbells. Your legs move through a full range of motion to blast your quads, glutes, and hamstrings.

Place your arms in the fighting position with your elbows in, hands up, and chin down. Hold a dumbbell in each hand. Stand with your feet slightly farther than shoulder's-width apart; point the toes of both feet straight ahead. Bend your knees until your thighs are parallel to the floor. Don't bend your knees too far. Move 3 seconds down and 3 seconds up for 10 reps.

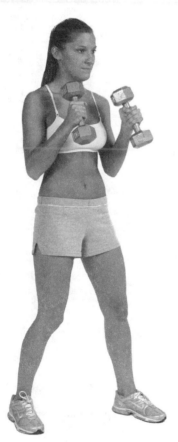

Keep your arms in close to your body simulating that you are wearing heavy boxing gloves.

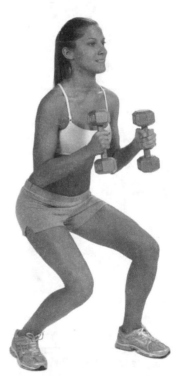

Squat only as far down as you feel comfortable while maintaining perfect posture.

Boxer's Lunge Lift

The Boxer's Lunge Lift provides a bonus buns training tool at the end of the move. When you lift your back leg, you fire all the muscles in your buns. This exercise is a great bun-shaper.

Start in a lunge position with your elbows in and hands up in a fighting stance. While holding a dumbbell in each hand, lift your back leg off the floor a few inches by contracting your hip. Balance for a second, lower, and then repeat the move for 10 reps.

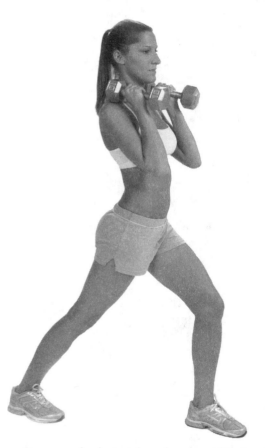

Keep your back straight rather than allowing the weights to pull you forward.

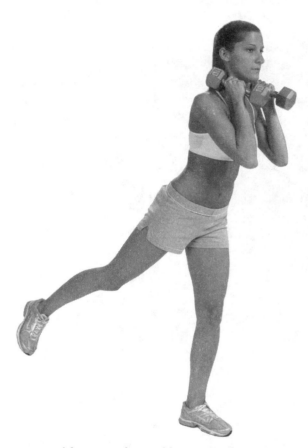

Bend from your hip and keep your chest out.

The Least You Need to Know

- Your legs are the foundation for every move you make. Train them correctly and they will serve you well.
- Lower-body training is hard. Mental preparation before doing a leg workout is essential.
- When you're first starting out, just lifting your own body weight might be enough resistance to provide you with a training effect. As you get stronger, add resistance (weights) to keep your muscles challenged.
- Your lower body muscles are larger than your upper body muscles. When you train your lower body, you're doing more work, which burns more calories.

In This Chapter

- ◆ The power of plyometrics
- ◆ Incorporating plyometrics into your exercise routine
- ◆ Making the jump
- ◆ Best plyometrics drills

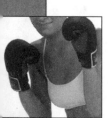
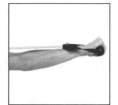
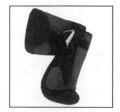
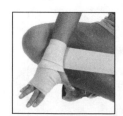
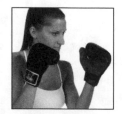
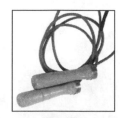

Floating Like a Butterfly

The great heavyweight boxer Muhammad Ali was noted for his unique boxing style, a combination of speed with devastating punching power that was described by one of his handlers as the ability to "float like a butterfly, sting like a bee."

Plyometrics are the key to developing that combination of power and speed. They're great for the ring, obviously, but the drills can do great things for your body, too. If you've ever admired the physique of a sprinter or a long jumper—especially their powerful, well-defined leg muscles—plyometrics can help you achieve them.

Jumping Around with Plyometrics

At first glance, *plyometrics* appear to be a bunch of jumping drills. At their most basic level, that's exactly what they are, but there's more to them than that. Plyometrics build both speed and strength by using your muscles' ability to stretch and recoil.

How? When you stretch a muscle beyond its resting length, the stretch reflex causes a rubberband-like response. This stretch reflex is your body's way of protecting yourself so you don't hurt your muscles. Rather than stretch a muscle until it tears, your muscle senses a stretch that is beyond resting length and then bounces back.

Plyometric drills harness this reflexive, elastic recoil. Doing them regularly will help you move faster than your normal rate of acceleration. You'll be able to throw a ball faster, hit a ball harder, and throw punches that are faster and more powerful. Plyometrics can also make your legwork movements quicker and help you stay light on your feet during your fitness boxing routines.

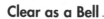

Clear as a Bell

Plyometrics are exercises that emphasize calisthenics and repeated movements such as jumping high off the ground. They're also known as jump training.

From a more technical, exercise physiology point of view, plyometric drills increase the size and activity of your fast-twitch muscle fibers. Fast-twitch fibers are larger and more powerful in comparison to your slow-twitch, endurance fibers. Fast-twitch fibers are recruited when you jump high or punch hard. This increases your muscle mass, strength, and power and helps you burn more calories, even at rest. Most elite power athletes include plyometrics in their training programs. A regular dose of them will do great things for you, too.

Doing Plyometic Routines

Some people think that all plyometric moves involve jumping, but this isn't the case at all. Bending and extending your knees quickly is a plyometric exercise.

However, most plyometric routines are cardiovascular intense, and they can be tough on the joints. For these reasons, there's an increased risk of injury with many types of plyometric training. If you do them, proceed with caution and stay away from moves that will put more stress on your muscles and joints than you can handle. Bounce lightly through each rep with a relaxed posture.

If possible, schedule a session or two with a trainer or coach who's well-versed in plyometrics so you can learn how to do them right from the get-go. Also don't do plyometrics right after a meal or before bedtime. Plyometrics is one of the most vigorous exercises in existence. Be sure you are both mentally and physically ready to perform.

The following is a sample plyometrics routine you might try. It takes about 30 minutes and includes three plyometrics intervals, each lasting about 30 seconds, interspersed with 5-minute recovery periods. The recovery phases prepare you for your next effort interval. Active recovery such as jogging in place also helps to circulate lactic acid and to convert it to energy for your next plyometric drill. If you perform it twice a week, you'll push your anaerobic threshold, burn lots of calories, and challenge all your energy systems. You'll get fitter, increase muscle mass, and your metabolism will accelerate so you'll burn more calories at rest.

> Warm up: Jog in place—5 minutes
>
> Skip with exaggerated knee lift and long stride—30 seconds
>
> Jog in place (recovery phase)—5 minutes
>
> Sprint, raising knees high—30 seconds
>
> Jog in place (recovery phase)—5 minutes
>
> Standing broad jump forward and backward—5 consecutive
>
> One-legged jump—10 forward on right leg, 10 forward on left leg
>
> Jump up and down 10 times as quickly as you can, keeping your feet as close to the ground as possible
>
> Jog in place (recovery phase)—5 minutes
>
> Cool down and stretch

Use the various plyometrics exercises in this chapter to vary your workout and keep your muscles in a state of anticipation.

Sweet Science

According to the American Council on Fitness, plyometric training dates back to the 1970s, where it was used in Eastern Europe to develop greater strength and power in Olympic athletes.

Squat Thrust

Squat Thrusts are a great full-body workout. You'll train the muscles in your legs and upper body, and if you do more than five repetitions, you'll also get a fantastic cardiovascular workout.

Stand with your feet shoulder-width apart. Bend forward hinging at your hip with your palms facing the floor and your back straight.

Squat until your thighs are parallel to the floor. Place your palms flat on the floor beside your feet. Place your hands on the floor and assume a push-up position. Keep your weight over your arms and kick your feet straight back so that you end up in a push-up position.

Do one push-up, then hop back into a squat and return standing up in preparation for your next rep. Do 10 repetitions with correct form.

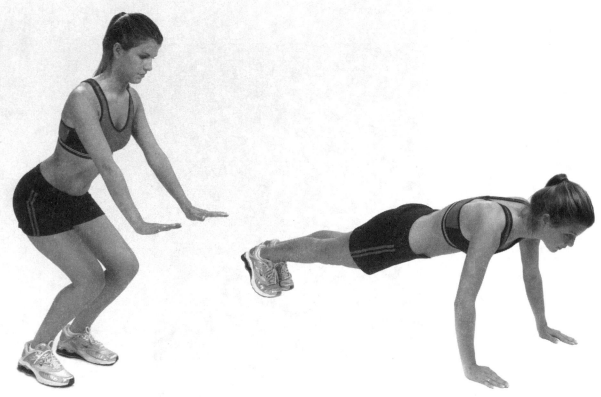

Squat Thrust starting position.   **Squat Thrust push-up position.**

🔘 Stair Sprint

Stair Sprints firm your thighs, buns, hamstrings, and calves. If you live in a house or apartment with a second floor, you've got it made. If not, you'll have to get creative and find some stairs to use.

This one couldn't be simpler. Just sprint up a flight of stairs. Take them one, two, or three at a time, depending on your fitness and comfort level. Pay attention to your form and watch your step. You don't want to fall. Keep your back straight and your head up. Try not to hunch forward to look at the stairs. Step as lightly as possible on each step and move quickly from step to step.

If the stairs are equipped with a handrail and you feel the need to use it, by all means do so. However, you'll get a better workout if you can swing your arms freely during this exercise.

Use your descent down the stairs as your rest period. When you get to the bottom, start back up again. Try to perform 10 repetitions. Be sure to maintain your form throughout each sprint.

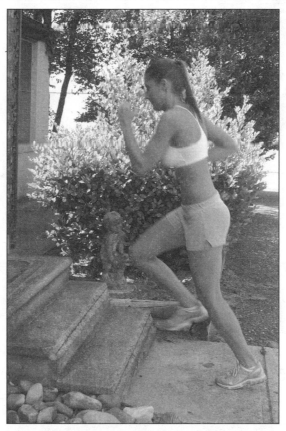

Keep your eyes focused a couple of steps ahead of you for balance.

Bunny Hop

This is a fun exercise that firms and tones all your leg muscles, and especially your calves. Try it with your kids—they'll love it!

Simply keep your legs together and jump forward about 3 inches. Bend your knees slightly and hop a few inches forward landing softly on the balls of your feet. Then jump back into start position. Rather than trying to hop far, try to take short, fast hops. Keep your hands up in a fighting position. Do 10 repetitions forward and backward with correct form.

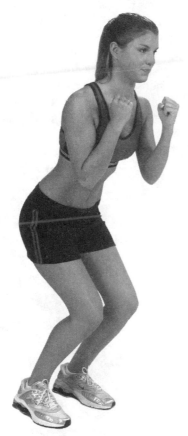

Bunny Hop start position.

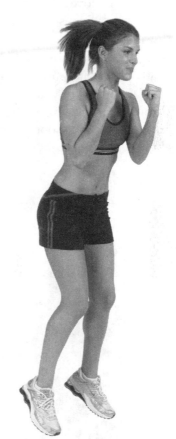

Make your hops short and fast.

Lateral Jump

Jumping from side to side firms and tones the muscles of your inner and outer thighs, and helps work the core muscles in your abs and back as you use them to stabilize your movement.

This is an intense move. Until your body gets accustomed to it, do just a few repetitions during each workout.

Begin with your feet shoulder-width apart and your hands up in a fighting position. Start by pressing off the inside of your left foot and jumping to your right foot. Continue jumping back and forth from foot to foot. Keep your back straight and your abs tight.

Rather than jumping high off of each foot, try more of a push—sliding back and forth attempting to achieve lateral speed rather than height. Do 10 repetitions side to side with correct form.

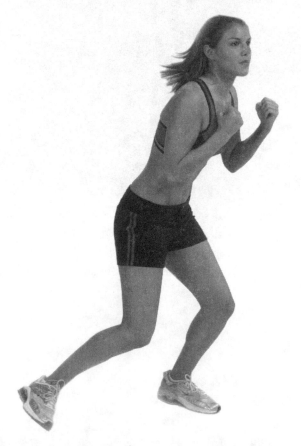

Knockout Punch

If you have any orthopedic problems or concerns, do one-legged exercises with both legs. Hopping on two feet requires less impact than hopping on one foot. Also perform plyometrics only if your joints are in great condition. Your ankles, knees, and back take quite a beating. If you are in doubt about the integrity of your joints, check with your physician before beginning a plyometric program.

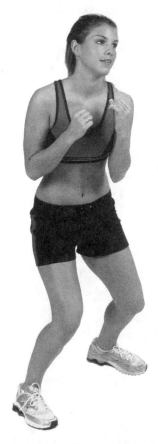

Starting position for Lateral Jumps.

Keep your movement horizontal instead of vertical.

One-Legged Jump Forward/Back

One-Legged Jumps forward and back stimulate the power muscles in your calves, thighs, buns, and hamstrings. They're great for defining and slimming your leg muscles.

Begin by standing on your left leg with your hands in the fighting position. Jump 3 inches forward and then 3 inches back. Switch legs and repeat with your right leg.

Jump fast instead of high or far. Stay on the ball of your foot. Try to land so softly that you barely make a sound. Do 10 repetitions forward and backward with correct form.

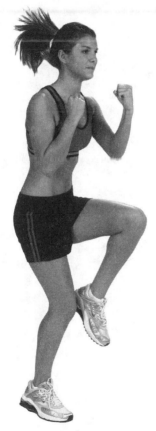

Keep your nonworking knee high for a more intense move.

Lunge Jump

The Lunge Jump focuses on toning your lower body muscles as well as the core muscles of your abs and back.

With your head up and back straight, step forward with your left leg. Lower your body until your front knee is bent 90 degrees and your right knee almost touches the floor. From this position, jump a few inches and switch feet in the air, landing with your other leg forward in the starting position.

Keep your hands up in the fighting position and maintain correct posture throughout each rep. Instead of trying to jump high, concentrate on switching the position of your feet, back and forth as quickly as you can. Do 10 repetitions with correct form, switching on each rep.

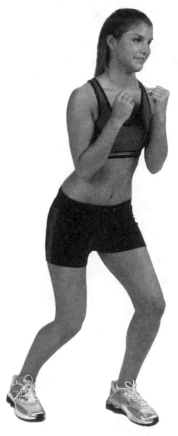

Lunge Jump starting position.

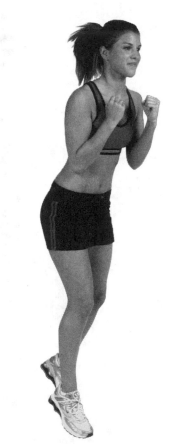

Midway through the Lunge Jump. Note the switch in foot position.

Alternate Knee

This plyometric move tones the muscles in your legs and buns and delivers a high-intensity cardiovascular workout at the same time.

Begin in a left leg forward fighting position. Drive your right knee into the air toward your chest while simultaneously jumping up with your left leg. Bring your left knee up toward your chest while straightening your right knee to land. Switch legs and repeat.

Jump an inch or two from the floor and maintain good posture throughout all your repetitions. Keep your hands up in the fighting position. Resist the temptation to drop your hands. Do 10 repetitions with correct form, switching on each rep.

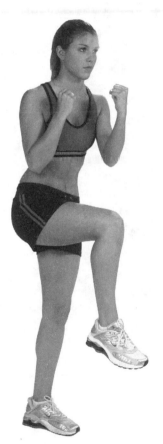
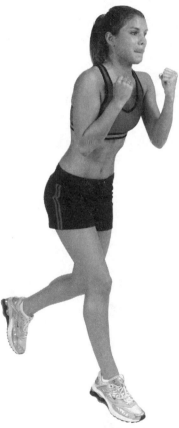
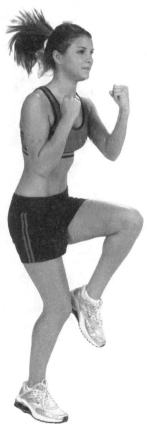

| Be sure to keep your knees high and your hands up. | Keep your legs straight but don't lock your knees when you land. | Jumps should be low and softly landed. |

Standing Long Jump

The Standing Long Jump works all the muscles in your lower body.

Stand with your feet less than shoulder-width apart and your hands in the fighting position. Flex your knees and jump forward as far as you can while keeping your hands in the fighting position. Do 10 repetitions with correct form.

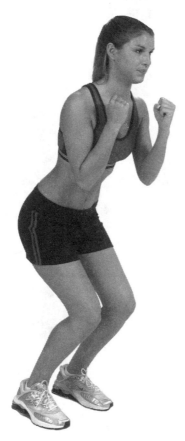

Standing Long Jump starting position.

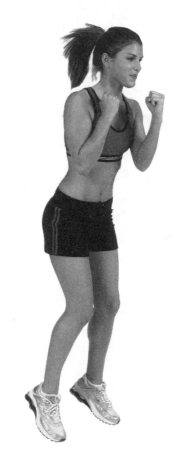

Keep your hands up and eyes focused ahead.

The Least You Need to Know

◆ Plyometrics develops the muscle's ability to stretch and recoil, just like a rubberband.

◆ You should be in good condition before attempting plyometrics. Your ankles, shins, knees, and hips should be pain-free if you intend to use plyometrics as part of your program.

◆ Be thoroughly warmed up before plyometric training. The warm up lubricates your joints and heats up your muscles for action.

◆ Plyometric exercises give you a great cardiovascular workout.

In This Part

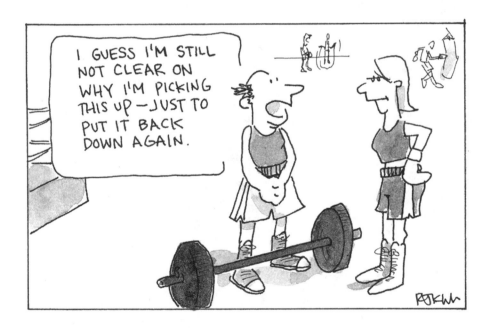

Building a Boxer's Body

Ever wonder why a boxer's body is so powerful looking and defined? Boxers don't spend endless hours in the weight room but they are ripped to the bone. From their streamlined calves to their rock-hard arms, they look great in and out of their clothes.

Part 2 teaches you to use all the toys that people in great shape consider a secret to getting a better body. Finally, if you're fortunate enough to convince a friend to work out with you, partner drills will motivate you to achieve the body of your dreams.

In This Chapter

- ◆ Staying motivated with training tools
- ◆ Protecting your hands and wrists
- ◆ Punching bags
- ◆ Timers
- ◆ Exercise bands and jump ropes
- ◆ Stability balls and medicine balls

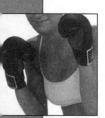
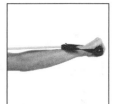
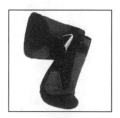
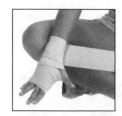
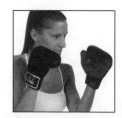
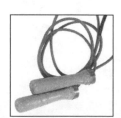

Chapter 5

Training Tools

Unlike some other types of exercise programs or regimens, you don't need a lot of equipment for fitness boxing. If you have basic exercise clothes and a good pair of workout shoes, you already have pretty much all you need.

That said, if you want to gear up and add some dash to your workouts, there are some training tools you can use for fitness boxing. They can help you keep motivated and can be used to measure your progress as you work your fitness boxing program.

In this chapter, we take a look at the various tools and toys that you can choose from to enhance your fitness boxing experience, and give you an idea of how they're used.

Hand and Wrist Protection

Even with good protection, hand injuries sideline more boxers than any other. Because there are so many small bones in your hand and wrist—30 of them, to be exact—it's absolutely imperative that you take every precaution available to protect them if you're going to include heavy bag and/or focus mitt work in your fitness boxing program.

Hand Wraps

Proper hand wrapping is the best way to prevent injury. Hand wraps, which are long strips of cloth, support the ligaments, bones, and muscles of your fists and cover your knuckles to keep your hands healthy for heavy bag training.

Sweet Science _____

You definitely don't need exercise toys to get in great shape, but they can sure help you stay motivated and help you stick to your exercise routine. You can purchase fitness boxing equipment at many sporting goods stores, martial arts supply companies, and on the Internet.

Hand wraps with Velcro are a good choice because they're easy to put on and easy to remove after a grueling workout. They cost less than $10 per pair—well worth the price for the protection they provide.

You might think that hand wraps are overkill, but they really aren't. Not only do they provide essential protection for the tiny bones in your hands and wrists, they pad the knuckles and give you the feeling of being a real boxer.

There are a variety of different ways to wrap your hands. Here's an easy approach that works well. If you're right handed, you might want to start with your left hand, but it really doesn't matter all that much:

1. Start by wrapping your wrist. Hold the hand you're going to wrap open and relaxed. Place the hand wrap in your palm and put your thumb through the thumb loop. Check to make sure that the "this side down" label is facing your palm. Start wrapping by going across the back of your hand first, then wrap three times around your wrist. Wrap it tight, but not so tight that it hampers your circulation.

2. Now that your wrist is braced, slide the wrap across the back of your hand and around your palm. Circle the wrap around your knuckles three times.

3. Wrap across the back of your hand toward your wrist three times in a figure 8 pattern across the back of your hand.

4. Continue around the palm of your hand toward your wrist. Fasten the hook and loop closure.

Repeat on the other hand and you're done. Your wrapped hands should be tight and secure, ready to rumble.

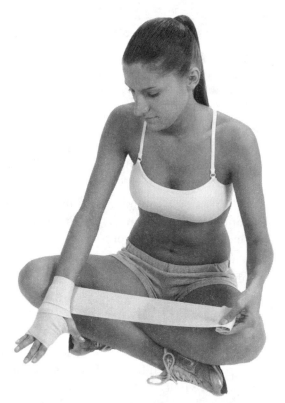

Wrap your wrists first, then your hands.

Gloves

Bag or training gloves are lighter and smaller than the gloves boxers use in the ring. Although they're padded, they don't have anywhere near the amount of padding that boxing gloves do. They weigh about 14 ounces and provide enough padding and support for hitting the heavy bag. They also slip on and off easily, unlike boxing gloves that have to be laced up. You wear bag gloves in addition to hand wraps.

Bag gloves come in various weights and styles. Some are designed especially to fit a women's hand. Fourteen-ounce leather bag gloves with Velcro wrist closures will cost you around $50.

Bag gloves are necessary when hitting the bag, but they are also fun to wear while training. They give you the feeling that you are a real boxer. They also add a couple of ounces of resistance to increase the intensity of your shadowboxing workout. (See Chapter 18 for some good shadowboxing workouts.)

Try different brands of bag gloves to find the style that suits your needs as they come in all different shapes and sizes. Some have more padding than others but the most important thing is to buy a brand that is washable. Your hands sweat more than you may think, so you will need to wash your bag gloves at least once a month depending on the frequency of your training.

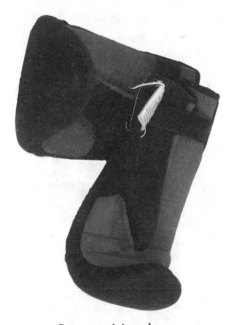

Bag or training gloves.

Focus Mitts

Focus mitts are gloves with an 8-inch diameter striking unit built around a shock-absorbing pad. They absorb the shock from punches, and are used when you train with a partner. Focus mitts for children or other special needs are also available.

A strap system holds the mitt firmly to the hand, which allows the holder of the mitts to relax. This reduces the chance of injury to the holder's arms and joints. Expect to spend around $45 for these.

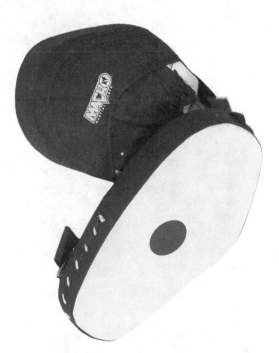

Use focus mitts when you train with a partner.

Heavy Bags

Heavy bags (or punching bags) are made of canvas, vinyl, or leather and contain fillings that are either soft or hard. There are even heavy bags that you can fill with water. Leather bags are the most durable and the most expensive, but canvas or nylon bags work just fine, too.

Prices for good quality, heavy bags range from $70 to $150.

Heavy bags come in various weights for different sports. For fitness boxing, you want a bag weighing around 70 pounds or so. Depending on the type of bag you buy, you'll need a stand, mounting attachments, and hanging equipment. If you're going to hang it in your house, you'll need to find a fairly substantial beam to hang it from. Or you can buy a freestanding heavy bag that sits on a round, weighted base. (You'll find heavy bag routines in Chapter 12.)

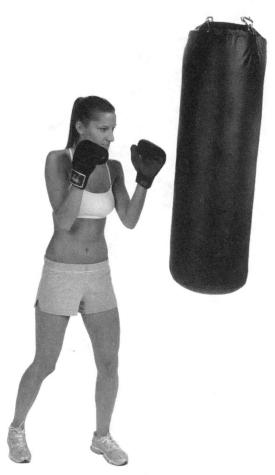

Heavy bag.

Knockout Punch

Some people like to do their heavy bag training outdoors, and put together a special setup so they can. This can be a lot of fun, but be sure not to leave your heavy bag up after you're done, especially if it might rain or snow. If the stuffing gets wet, it can weigh down the bag and tear the outside cover.

Timers

An egg timer not only tells you when to start and stop when you're doing intervals, it can also be a huge motivator. Think of it as a little coach—it won't give you any slack or be too easy on you. Give your best for 3 minutes; when you hear the "ding," you can relax for a minute. The feeling of relief and gratification when you hear that final bell can't be beat.

Egg timers are cheap and widely available. That said, even if you already have one, you might want to upgrade to a fancier model that will let you time three different activities at once—you can use the three different alarms for different rounds.

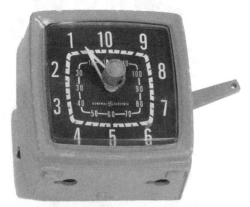

This model can be programmed to time three different activities at once.

A cheap timer shouldn't cost you more than $10. Expect to spend another $5 or so for fancier models.

Exercise Bands

Exercise bands are made of synthetic materials such as carbon polymers, polyvinyl chloride, fiberglass, or rubber. As the elastic stretches, the resistance increases. This challenges your muscles more as you reach the end range of the motion. Because exercise bands follow the line of pull of your muscle, they tone your muscles at angles that other devices can't. (You'll find band training routines in Chapter 14.)

As part of a fitness boxing program, exercise bands add consistency, strength, and power to your movements. They also help you develop explosive strength, which is necessary for getting the most benefit from your punches.

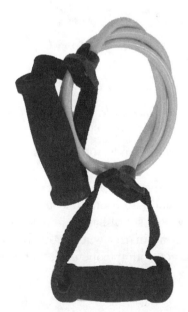

Exercise band.

Exercise bands come in various styles—tubes, flat, with handles, and without handles. The simplest ones work as well, if not better than the fancy ones.

The color of the band indicates the resistance level. You can also increase resistance by shortening the length of the band, either by folding it up in your hand or by moving your feet around.

Exercise bands are great for keeping up your fitness boxing routine when you travel. They take up virtually no space in your luggage, and you can use them just about anywhere.

Bands are fairly durable when used properly. Be sure to keep them out of direct sun, and check them regularly for wear and tear. Look for changes in tension, splits, and cracks in both the band and the handles.

Exercise bands are inexpensive and available at large discount stores as well as on the Internet at www.spriproducts.com. If possible, buy several bands of various resistances—light, medium, and heavy—or buy a package that contains all three.

Sweet Science

Using an exercise band allows you to train at any speed through both the lifting and lowering phase. This means that you can firm your muscles, burn a lot of calories, and get a great workout in a short period of time.

Jump Ropes

The best exercise devices are simple and inexpensive. This one fits in your suitcase and is so easy your children can do it better than you. But don't fool yourself. Jump ropes are not just for kids. Professional boxers are fantastic rope skippers, and there are lots of good reasons why such a simple tool is such a big part of their workouts, including the following:

◆ It improves agility, coordination, rhythm, and timing.

◆ It helps build explosive power.

◆ It's easy on the joints. When you jump, you bounce lightly on the balls of your feet and your calves absorb the shock.

◆ It's great for strengthening your heart.

What's more, jumping rope is a fantastic calorie burner. If you're of average weight and average fitness, you can burn 150 calories in just 10 minutes of jumping rope nonstop.

Different types of ropes provide different workouts. Speed jumpers use thin ropes while competitive double-dutch trick ropers use thicker cloth ropes. There are also jump ropes with weighted handles, but you really don't need them to get a great workout. Instead, look for a medium-weight leather or plastic rope. A beaded thin rope, strung with half-inch plastic beads, also works well for fitness boxing. The beads help the rope swing evenly and consistently. Plan to spend around $15 for a beaded rope. Stay away from light, cotton ropes—they aren't dense enough to swing around your head and feet unless you go really fast.

Your height determines the length of your rope. If you're between 5'4" and 5'10", use a nine-foot rope. If you're between 5'11" and 6'6", a 10-foot rope is best. If you're taller than 6'6", you'll need an 11-foot rope. If you're under 5'4", try adjusting a short rope to fit or buying a children's rope. When you step in the center of the rope, the handles should barely reach your armpits. The rope should barely brush the floor when you jump. If it doesn't touch the floor, it's too short. If it drags on the floor, it's too long.

Corner Man _____

Try it before you buy it. Wear workout clothes and try your jump rope, exercise band, medicine ball, stability ball, and heavy bag before making an investment. If the store will not let you try before you buy, go to another store.

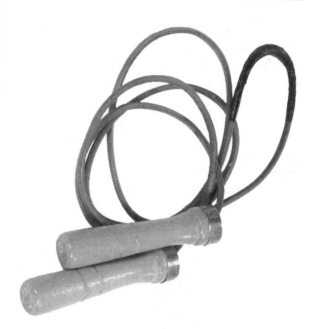

Inexpensive plastic ropes spin the fastest.

Like exercise bands, jump ropes are great for keeping up your fitness boxing program when you're traveling. They're light, portable, and take up virtually no room in a suitcase. Throw a rope in with a set of bands, and you'll be able to work out no matter where you are. (You'll find some good jump rope drills in Chapter 2.)

Stability Balls

When you exercise on a stability ball, one set of muscles contracts to balance your body while opposing muscle groups lengthen. This results in a much greater training effect, as you have to use your muscles to perform the exercises and to remain balanced.

Stability balls come in various shapes and styles. In general, it's best to choose a round ball over oblongs or the type with small feet on the bottom, as they're the most versatile. Oblongs are easier to balance on, but if you're having trouble balancing, just letting some air out of a round ball will help. Balls with feet stay in place, which pretty much defeats the purpose of stability balls.

Corner Man

If you already own a stability ball but it's too large, just let some air out. If it's too small, you're better off buying a new one.

You'll want to choose the right ball to fit your height. When you sit on the ball, your feet should touch the ground and your knees should be flexed at a 90-degree angle. If you're shorter than 5'4", buy a ball that's 55cm, or 21 to 22 inches in diameter. If you're 5'5" to 5'11", buy a 65cm (25 to 26 inches) ball. Taller than 5'11", choose a 75cm (29 to 30 inches) ball. Good stability balls run anywhere from $20 to $40.

More ball-buying pointers:

◆ Choose a burst-resistant ball. If punctured, these balls release air slowly instead of bursting suddenly.

◆ Buy a pump. A bike pump will work (you might need an adapter, which your ball should come with), but a small pump designed for inflating these balls is handy, not to mention a good workout on their own!

◆ Get a plug puller. Stability ball plugs are designed to stay in place, which makes them hard to remove. A plug puller will save you lots of time and effort, and will make it easier to take your ball with you when you travel.

Like exercise bands, stability balls are fairly durable. However, they can get scratched up and dirty. If you need to wash your ball, use a mild detergent. Harsh chemicals will break them down. So will direct sunlight and chlorine. If you have a pool and you like to workout outside, you might want to think twice about adding exercise bands and a stability ball to the mix. (You'll find stability ball drills in Chapter 8.)

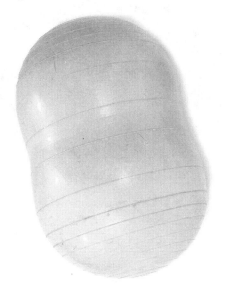

Stability ball.

Medicine Balls

Medicine balls are kind of an old-fashioned training tool, but they're still with us for a good reason: they work! Like exercise bands, when you throw the ball, you train your muscles at all different angles and speeds. Plus, training with a medicine ball more closely resembles punching than lifting weights does. When you throw a medicine ball or throw a punch, you don't slow down your movement at the end, like you do when you lift weights. Instead, you keep moving throughout the movement.

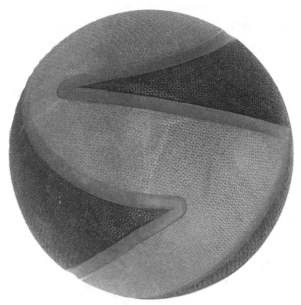

Medicine ball.

Medicine balls can also train your nervous system to explode through a movement by using your fast-twitch speed and power muscle fibers. Finally, another advantage of medicine ball training is that it develops both sides of your body. You learn to throw and catch with both arms just as in fitness boxing where you learn to jab and hook with your left, throw a cross with your right, and uppercut with both arms. Medicine ball training is as great as throwing punches because it simulates the muscle activity required to follow through on a punch. Punching is more like throwing a ball than lifting a weight. You don't decelerate when throwing a punch; instead, your goal is to hit through to your target. When throwing a medicine ball, you don't slow down your throw at the end range of motion. When lifting weights, you do slow down your movement at the end range of motion.

Medicine balls come in different shapes, sizes, and colors. Today's medicine balls are made of durable rubber compounds that last for years. Some medicine balls have a full bounce which is great for outdoor use. Indoor versions have little or no bounce so you can work safely in a confined area. You can get med balls ranging from 2 to 8 pounds from $20 to $40 per ball.

Start with a light, small ball that you can easily handle for every drill. As you progress in skill and strength, you can use heavier balls. (You'll find medicine ball drills in Chapter 7.)

For more information on medicine balls, go to Power Systems at www.power-systems.com or Perform Better at www.performbetter.com/.

The Least You Need to Know

◆ You don't need special training tools to get in great shape, but they can help keep you motivated and take you to the next level of fitness.

◆ In fitness boxing, your hands and wrists are especially prone to injury; make sure you protect them with wraps, gloves, or mitts.

◆ A punching bag is the best training partner because it never has an excuse and is always on time. Punching a bag improves your speed and power, and increases your strength and muscle tone.

◆ A timer is your personal trainer. It tells you when to start and stop. Wait for that final "ding" before heading for the shower.

◆ Bands and jump ropes are inexpensive and versatile tools that tone and strengthen your body. They are so lightweight and compact that you can use them at the office or when you travel.

◆ Stability balls and medicine balls are exercise toys that make your workout effective and fun.

In This Chapter

◆ Locating classes

◆ Selecting the right instructor

◆ Tips on what to wear

◆ Pre-class do's and don'ts

◆ What to expect in a class

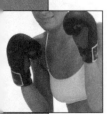
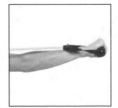
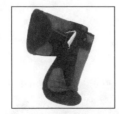
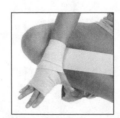
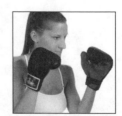
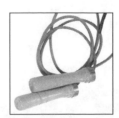

Chapter 6

Boxing in a Class

Fitness boxing is a great do-it-yourself workout, but it's also fantastic in a class setting. Not only do you have the camaraderie of those around you as you jump rope, shadowbox, bob, weave, and shuffle your way to a brand-new body, there's music to inspire your punches and blocks, too. And when there's a group of people punching in perfect unison to a driving beat, the hard work just seems a little easier.

Participating in fitness boxing classes is also a great way to learn how to do the moves the right way. If you're thinking about taking some classes, this chapter will tell you what to expect.

Finding Fitness Boxing Classes

This one's pretty easy. If you belong to a health club or other type of exercise facility, check the class roster. Chances are good there's at least a fitness boxing class or two on it. If you don't belong to a club, you'll probably be able to find classes at community centers, gyms, and boxing gyms.

If possible, choose a class that matches your experience and fitness level. That said, if the offerings are "one size fits all," they can still work for you, and you'll find suggestions on tailoring them to fit your needs later in this chapter.

Knockout Punch _____

Signing up for a series of fitness boxing classes might seem like a good idea, and it can be if the classes are on a reasonable schedule—say two or three times a week at the most—and if the schedule is flexible, meaning that you can go at your own pace and don't have to finish the series in a prescribed time period. Taking classes more than two or three days a week, especially in the beginning, can lead to overtraining and/or injury. Avoid any facility or program that calls for more than this.

Before you participate in a class, you might be asked to fill out a health-risk appraisal questionnaire to assess your general health and fitness level. As discussed in Chapter 1, it's always a good idea to consult with a physician and get a physical before embarking on any fitness program. It's especially important to do so if any of the following conditions apply:

◆ Adult older than 35

◆ Sedentary for a long period of time

◆ High blood pressure or other heart-related concern

◆ Recent surgeries

◆ Pregnant

◆ Taking medications that regulate heart rate

◆ Any other medical conditions that intense workouts could negatively affect

None of these conditions mean you can't take fitness boxing classes, but they might call for additional modifications that should be discussed with the instructor and your doctor.

Choosing an Instructor

Fitness boxing's popularity means you have a choice in instructors. Take advantage of this and choose wisely, as a good instructor can make a big difference in your progress.

One of the best ways to pick good instructors is to watch them teach. Watching a fitness boxing class is best, but you can get an idea of the instructor's style regardless of class format. Most instructors will let you watch or try a class before enrolling.

A good instructor should do the following:

◆ Watch everyone's form and make corrections when necessary.

◆ Develop rapport with students.

◆ Monitor heart rates and/or perceived exertion periodically throughout the workout so intensity can be individualized to needs.

◆ Readily discontinue her workout during class to correct form and/or answer questions. She should be concerned with her students' workout, not her own.

◆ Adjust the intensity of the workout according to the needs of the class.

◆ Demonstrate techniques carefully and thoroughly, first slow, then to speed.

Different instructors have different teaching styles, which may or may not fit what you prefer. Previous competitive boxing experience is helpful but not necessary. That said, a teacher who has a background in the ring probably won't waste your time with grapevines and other cute aerobic moves, and if they're not to your liking either, it could be a good fit. Instructors with no boxing experience might be a little heavy on the choreography.

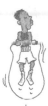

Sweet Science _____

Instructors who hold a nationally recognized fitness certification can help you with questions regarding your diet, stress management, and many other fitness topics. They're also required to stay current on their cardiopulmonary resuscitation (CPR) certification.

Find someone else to take classes from if you see any of the following:

◆ Class members not being able to keep up with the moves. Instructors should match the workout to meet the needs of the class, not the other way around. A good instructor trains you according to your needs and fitness level. A "no pain is gain" philosophy keeps you coming back again and again.

◆ Instructors verbally "beating up" on class participants. This is an older "drill sergeant" style of instruction, and definitely not necessary. You might think you'd benefit from the drill instructor approach, but a commandant style wears thin after about a week for just about everyone.

◆ Instructors who make students perform multitudes of complicated, choreographed drills. Drills like this aren't any more effective than simpler moves are.

◆ Instructors who leave immediately after the class is over. They should hang around for a few minutes both before and after class to answer questions or offer extra coaching.

◆ Students sweating profusely and barely able to walk out of the gym. Some "old school" teachers think it's a badge of honor to work their students to utter exhaustion by the end of a class. They think wrong.

The best instructors are empathetic, genuine, and warm. They listen to your goals and effectively teach you how to reach them. They're good role models and they demonstrate exemplary form for each drill. They motivate you and provide you with feedback concerning your form. Finally, they should be willing to spend some extra time with you to answer your questions and help you with your form.

Sweet Science

If you do find a great instructor, and want to keep her, be sure to let the manager of the club know what a great job she's doing.

Finally, instructors should be certified by a national organization such as the American Council on Exercise (ACE), American College of Sports Medicine (ACSM), the National Strength and Conditioning Association (NSCA), or the Aerobic and Fitness Association of America (AFAA). The facility should readily make these certifications available for all instructors. If they're withheld for any reason, find somewhere else to train.

What to Wear

Loose fitting, comfortable, breathable clothing is a necessity for fitness boxing. The last thing you want to do is wear anything that hampers your movement, so leave the tight spandex at home. Good choices include the following:

◆ **Short-sleeved or sleeveless tops.** Choose a breathable fabric, such as Cool Max, that wicks moisture away from your skin. Cotton retains moisture, and gets heavier as it does—even thin cotton t-shirts will do this.

◆ **Workout shorts or pants.** Again, choose a breathable fabric that wicks moisture away from your skin. Make sure your shorts or pants are loose enough to let you move freely. Crop pants or capris are a good choice if you want a little more coverage than shorts provide but also want to stay a little cooler as you're working out.

◆ **Sports bra.** For the girls, obviously. Pick a good one that provides support similar to what you'd need if you were running or taking an aerobic dance class. Again, choose a material that won't weigh you down when you work up a sweat.

Basic cross training or aerobic training shoes will work fine. Whatever you wear needs to allow you to pivot on the balls of your feet. Socks should also be made of synthetic material that wicks the moisture away from your feet.

A few more tips:

◆ If your hair is long, tie it back.

◆ Don't wear strong perfume or cologne—working out hard in close quarters tends to intensify aromas.

◆ If you don't bring your own equipment to class, be prepared to use one-size-fits-all gloves that might still be sweaty from the last person who used them. As mentioned in Chapter 5, practice gloves vary from 8 to 16 ounces. The heavier the glove, the harder the workout. When you're just starting out, you'll probably want to select the lightest gloves unless you're already in fairly good shape. You want to make it through the class, not impress anyone with the size of your gloves.

◆ Always bring your own hand wraps (see Chapter 5).

Pre-Class Prep

Get to your class a few minutes early so you can warm up on your own. There's nothing worse than rushing into a class that's already started, or even half over, and injuring yourself because you missed the warm-up.

Come mentally prepared. Rather than rush to class without any forethought, practice some of the moves in your mind so that they will be easier to execute.

If permitted, take the equipment for a test drive before the class begins. If you're going to hit the heavy bag, take the time to put on your hand wraps. Don't worry about being a rank beginner and looking silly; remember that everyone starts at the same level. The people in your class who look like pros once felt as awkward as you do.

Bring a bottle of water. Sip regularly instead of running back and forth to the water fountain.

Bring two towels. One is for wiping sweat from your eyes, face, and anywhere else you need it. The other is to wipe down the floor and any equipment you use as a courtesy to others.

Your meal schedule will affect both your attitude during class and how you fare physically during the class. If your muscles aren't fueled properly, you might be irritable. You also might feel sluggish and tired, which is definitely not conducive to a quality workout.

If it's been several hours since your last meal, a light snack prior to class is a good idea. Also pack an energy bar in your workout bag to munch on should you become shaky or light headed during class and need an extra boost.

Knockout Punch

Be careful not to eat a huge meal anytime near your class. Doing so can make you feel lethargic as your body needs to focus its energy on digestion. Eating or drinking too much before class might also make you feel a bit queasy.

Inside a Fitness Boxing Class

No two fitness boxing classes are ever alike, but there are basic elements and moves that are common to most of them.

Most fitness boxing classes last for around 60 minutes and begin with a series of basic warm-up moves, such as wide-stance deep breaths, shoulder rolls, and light upper body twists to slow music without a beat.

Next the instructor might move into lower body marches in place, side steps, and other footwork patterns. After your lower body is sufficiently warmed up, you'll progress into conditioning moves such as upper body moves, including jabs and other punch combinations. These exercises focus on muscle strength and endurance, speed, and anaerobic conditioning. They're all performed with music, but you don't have to stay with the beat.

The heart of the workout will be intense activity intervals that might include rope jumping, working on the heavy bag, hitting focus mitts, and more. A one-minute active recovery period will follow each interval.

Corner Man

It's easy to be overzealous when you begin your training and overdo things. Inform your instructor that you are a beginner so he or she can point out breaks in your form.

Finally, there will be a cool down period, during which you'll do lower intensity exercises and stretches designed to bring your heart rate down and allow your body to recover.

Moving to the Music

Just about all fitness boxing classes are accompanied by music. Fitness boxing music is energizing, and it's a blast to perform boxing drills to the beat of your favorite tunes. In fact, some of your classmates are there *just* for the music.

Fitness boxing music plays at around 118 to 135 beats per minute (bpm). Warm-up tempos range from 120 to 125 bpm. The actual aerobic workout segment will be at anywhere from 125 to 134 bpm. Cool down tempos range from 118 to 122 bpm.

When you perform your fitness boxing drills, you can decide how hard you want to work out by matching your moves to the beat. Here's how:

◆ For a slow, easy workout, count two beats for each move (step, punch, and so on).

◆ For a medium-fast workout, count one beat for each move.

◆ For a fast-paced workout, move double-time, such as two punches per beat.

Or you can move to your own beat. Remember you aren't required to move to the beat at all; it's your option.

If this is confusing, just ask your instructor for help. He or she will be able to show you how to find the beat and how to match it to your ability and fitness levels.

If you can't move with the fast beat, or you cannot follow the choreography, just walk through the movements at an easy pace. Each subsequent class will be easier to follow.

Working the Circuits

Your class might include various training circuits. Pairing up with another classmate to punch the heavy bag is a common one. You might begin with a combination such as a jab, cross while your partner holds the bag. Then switch places and your partner does the same routine while you hold the bag and catch your breath.

You may do the same with focus mitts. You hold the mitts while your partner hits them and then you switch. Your rest period is the time you are holding the mitts.

Your instructor may also allow you to shadow spar with each other. These are pre-arranged moves where you know what your partner is going to do in advance. For example she may throw a jab and you slip her jab. Or you may throw a cross and she performs a duck under. You will learn these moves in other chapters and they should be done with plenty of margin for error. Your instructor should be circulating through the room to help you with your form.

Pairing Up

Some fitness boxing classes put more of an emphasis on pairing up to work out than others do, but just about all of them include some partner work. It can be fun to work out with your friends and enjoy the camaraderie as well as the built-in motivation that working out with others provide. However, it's not for everyone. If you're more the solitary type, don't ditch the class when you're instructed to pair up. Stick with it. Not only will you miss out on some good training if you don't, you might miss the chance to meet someone you like.

When working out with a partner, be sure not to measure your progress based on the other person's fitness level, skills, and abilities. Encourage her instead, and let her encourage you.

Staying Safe

Knowing how hard you're working is key to a safe, effective workout. You don't want to push so hard that you put your health at risk, but you also don't want to hold back so much that you're barely exerting yourself at all.

In most fitness classes, exertion is measured on something called the perceived exertion (PE) scale, which is a 1 to 10 ranking of—you guessed it—how hard you think you're working. A 1 means that you are barely working. A 10 signifies that you're working so hard that you can barely breathe.

Your instructor should stop periodically and ask you to assess your perceived exertion level, both to protect against problems and to modify the intensity of the workout to meet your needs. When you're first starting out, you'll want to keep it a little low, especially if you're not in shape. As you get more fit, you'll be able to work out safely at higher levels.

Here are some tips for staying safe and making the most of your class:

◆ Keep your knees soft (slightly bent). This protects your joints and reduces back strain.

◆ Limit high-intensity moves. Anything more than one-minute intervals is going too fast for too long and will burn you out.

◆ Limit repeater moves to 10 at a time. Vary your position periodically when doing them to prevent overuse injuries.

◆ Don't hold hand weights unless you're in very good shape. The few extra calories you might burn aren't worth it and increase the risk of injury.

◆ Never pivot on your weight-bearing leg. Doing so can blow out your knee. Be sure to shift your weight before doing the move.

◆ Always substitute a low-intensity move for a high-intensity move that's too difficult. If you need help, ask your instructor.

◆ Never hold your breath. It's common for new fitness boxing enthusiasts to hold their breath on punches. Instead, remind yourself to exhale at the completion of each punch. Doing so will let you work out longer and harder without fatigue.

◆ Keep talking to a minimum. Not only does it disturb other students, it takes your focus away from what you're doing, which can lead to injury. Save chatting for before and after class.

◆ Don't be anxious. Everybody feels a little nervous when they first begin taking a class because they don't know what to expect. You'll feel like a pro within a month.

◆ Be sure to move at your pace, not your instructor's. Your comrades may have been punching for years, so be patient with your progress.

◆ Be careful about how much space you're taking up in your fitness boxing room. Sometimes in a crowded class, you may be punching down the back of your classmate's neck and not even realize it.

◆ Don't stay in the back of the room because you're intimidated by your classmates. Work your way up into the second or third row where the instructor can see you and correct your form, and you can see him or her better to follow the moves.

Last but not least, focus on mastering a few basic skills during each class. Focus on training rather than fretting over intricate step combinations.

The Least You Need to Know

◆ If you are a beginner and looking for a fitness boxing class, watch a few classes and decide if you like the temperament and teaching style of the instructor. Also, talk to some of the students to find out their favorite choices of classes and instructors.

◆ Choose your instructor just as you would choose your doctor or dentist. Is he good at what she does? Is she willing to spend time explaining difficult techniques to you?

◆ Wear comfortable, loose-fitting, breathable clothing to your fitness boxing class. If the air conditioning is on overdrive, dress in layers and remove them as your body temperature increases.

◆ Before you walk into the exercise studio take a few minutes to mentally prepare for your workout. Once inside the studio, move through some of the basic punches and footwork using the mirror to check your form.

◆ Always err on the side of working out too easy rather than too hard. Concentrate on your form and stay relaxed.

In This Chapter

◆ Build strength (and have fun!) with a medicine ball

◆ What's involved in a basic medicine ball workout

◆ Throwing and catching

◆ Partnering with the ball

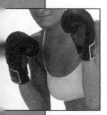 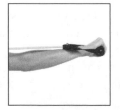 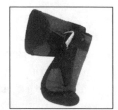 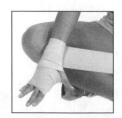 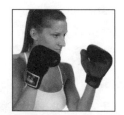 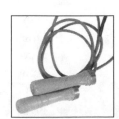

Chapter 7

Powering Up with Power Balls

Exercise doesn't have to be tedious or intense to be effective, and working with a medicine or power ball will drive this point home real fast.

Tossing around a heavy ball—which is all that a medicine ball is—may seem more like recreation than a great workout, but don't fool yourself for a minute. It's a very effective way to build muscle strength and size or just tone muscles, if that's your goal. Beyond this, medicine ball training is just plain fun!

Building Strength Through Speed and Resistance

Medicine or med ball training is strength training with a twist. Like other strength training approaches, it builds muscle strength and size, but instead of doing it the traditional way—by increasing reps, sets, or loads—it does it through a unique combination of speed and resistance.

Sound confusing? Technically, you're working on increasing your power by increasing your speed of movement. The good thing is, you don't really have to understand why it works. Just know that it does!

Tossing a medicine ball around works muscles at different speeds and angles. This not only gives you a great workout, it also helps increase your balance, your reaction time, and your agility, too.

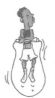

Med ball training uses explosive strength— you'll contract your muscles forcefully and use a greater percentage of powerful fast-twitch rather than slow-twitch endurance fibers— which means you'll exert maximal force in minimal time. Doing this well calls for being rested and refreshed, both physically and mentally. Be sure you're fully recovered from any previous activity before doing medicine ball workouts. Doing so will allow you to better concentrate on your moves, which, in turn, will allow you to get more out of them.

If you've never used medicine balls before, simply start by playing catch, either with yourself or with a partner. Or you can jump right into the following drills. After several months, start increasing the speed of your throws. Concentrate on simulating the act of punching as closely as you can when you throw.

If you don't have a partner, you can throw the ball against a wall, a heavy bag, or a rebounder. (A rebounder is a trampoline-like device that faces you at about a 45-degree angle from the ground. You can change the angle depending how fast you throw the ball at it.)

Hold the ball with both hands to minimize tendon and ligament stress. Be careful not to rear back and heave the ball with one hand. Be sure to maintain correct form throughout the range of motion.

As you get in better shape, challenge yourself by throwing the ball faster. And as you get stronger, increase the weight of the ball. Just as you would increase the weight of your dumbbells when an exercise becomes easy, the same applies with the med ball.

Basic Medicine Ball Workout

Here's a sample 30-minute medicine ball workout that you can do twice a week. Be sure to vary the program from time to time by switching the medicine ball exercises it contains with others in this chapter. Try not to rest at all between segments.

> Warm up: Slow shadowboxing— 5 minutes
>
> Bob and Weaver—2 minutes
>
> Jump Rope, Propellers—3 minutes
>
> Crouch Openers—2 minutes
>
> Jump Rope, Skier—3 minutes
>
> Torso Tightener—5 minutes
>
> Jump Rope, Figure 8s—3 minutes
>
> The Twist—2 minutes
>
> Cool down: Slow shadowboxing— 4 minutes; Arms Up Stretch—1 minute (hold onto the medicine ball and stand and reach up as high as you can with both arms over your head)

Bob and Weaver

This exercise, which mimics the motions of chopping wood, works most of the torso muscles, including your abdominal obliques and your lower back. It's also a good stretch for these muscles.

Hold onto the medicine ball with both hands. Raise the ball above your head, rotating the ball to your right. Inhale as you do. Bring it down on a diagonal pattern, close to your left knee. Exhale as you bring the ball down from your shoulder toward your knee.

Alternate the wood-chopping motion from left to right. Move slowly through the range of motion until the movement feels natural.

Keep your movements small and subtle at first. Then when you're ready for a challenge, increase your amplitude with wider, more expressive movements.

Knockout Punch

Keeping the muscles around your spine strong and flexible prevents back pain, but be sure to check with your doctor if you have any problems that might prevent you from doing some of the medicine ball exercises. Don't attempt any bending and twisting movements with the medicine ball; this will increase the risk of a back injury.

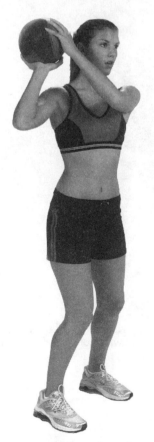

Starting position for Bob and Weaver.

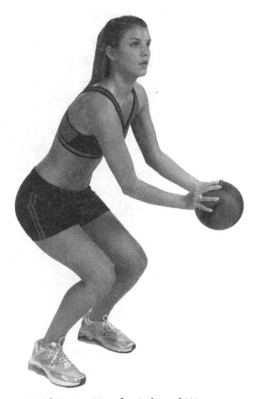

Finishing position for Bob and Weaver.

Crouch Opener

This exercise is a great stretch for your abs. When you stretch your abs and then flex them, you are fully working these muscles to get them firm and toned. It's also good for the back, as you extend your spine with each repetition. You'll need a partner for this exercise.

Lift the ball overhead and bend back slightly to stretch and strengthen the stomach muscles. Extend your back until you feel a stretch in your stomach muscles, then toss the ball to your partner a couple of feet away from you. The partner catches and throws it back, forcing you to reach up. The movement strengthens your arms and abs. Be careful to move slowly and gracefully.

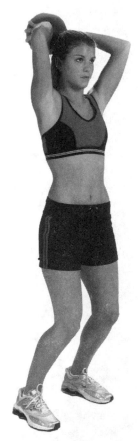

Crouch Opener starting position.

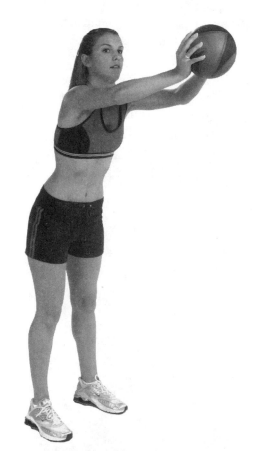

Keep your elbows soft and flex your back forward as you throw with both hands to your partner.

Torso Tightener

The Torso Tightener firms your upper body muscles and improves your hand-eye coordination and rhythm.

Stand facing your partner, a couple of feet apart. Squat, leaning forward at a slight angle.

Keep your knees bent, back straight, and eyes up. Pull your abdomen tight and toss the ball underhand on a diagonal pattern. You want to achieve a rotating motion. Toss the ball slowly to your partner, aiming for his or her hands. Your partner should squat down and catch it low.

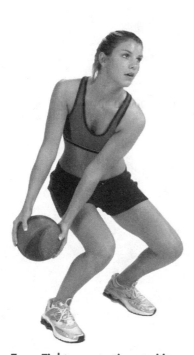

Torso Tightener starting position.

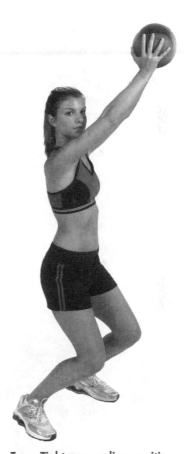

Torso Tightener ending position.

Boxer's Partner Sit-Up

Boxer's Partner Sit-Ups are the quintessential ab exercise. They train your abs at a full range of motion and use different speeds and angles to target all your abdominal muscle fibers. Be prepared for some tenderness with this one—it challenges everyone!

Ideally, you should have a training partner for this one. If you don't, you'll need to hook your feet under something to hold them in position.

Assume a bent knee sit-up position on the stability ball or the floor. Have your training partner stand on your feet to hold them down.

Lift your shoulder blades no higher than a few inches off the floor. Now have your partner throw the medicine ball to you so you can catch it at chest level. Allow the force from the impact to push you almost to the floor. Just before your back touches, sit up forcefully and toss the ball back to your partner with both hands.

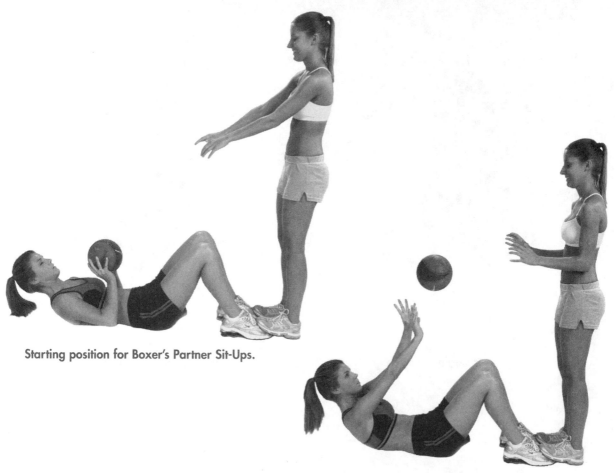

Starting position for Boxer's Partner Sit-Ups.

When you throw the ball back, lean forward and contract your ab muscles.

Crunch and Stretch

This move works all your ab, chest, and back muscles. It's more difficult than Boxer's Partner Sit-Ups as it calls for extending your arms over your head, which increases the intensity. It's another one that works best with a training partner, but if you can find something to anchor your feet under, you should be fine.

Assume a bent knee sit-up position on the stability ball or on the floor. Have a training partner stand on your feet to hold them down.

Begin sitting up with your back straight. Hold both arms outstretched over your head. Have your partner pass the ball lightly into your hands. Keeping your arms over your head, let the weight of the ball pull you back a few inches. To protect your back, only rock back an inch or two when you catch the ball. Then sit up straight and pass the ball back to your partner.

 ## Corner Man

Dynamic stretching, or what occurs in the Crunch and Stretch, builds flexible strength, meaning you'll have the strength to handle your newfound flexibility.

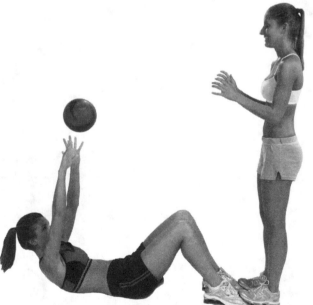

Crunch and Stretch starting position.

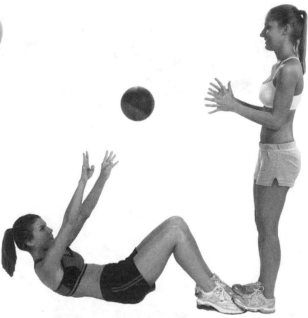

When you throw the ball, you should feel your chest and stomach muscles stretch and contract.

The Twist

All your ab muscles fire when you do this exercise, and the sides of your stomach will feel it for days. It's a great one for improving the upper body twisting power in your punches.

Assume a sit-up position on the stability ball or on the floor with your feet locked under a stationary object or with a partner holding them down. Sit up at a 45-degree angle to the floor. Hold a medicine ball in both hands straight out from your face. Keep your arms bent slightly.

Twist your torso rhythmically from side to side. Concentrate on twisting to one side, suddenly reversing the momentum, and twisting to the other side. The emphasis is on the obliques, shoulder, and lower back.

If the exercise is too difficult with your arms extended, try it from a bent-arm position.

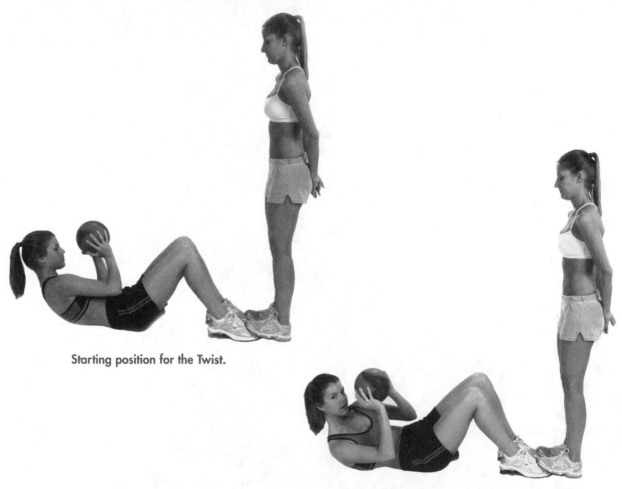

Starting position for the Twist.

Twist only far enough to feel a light stretch and then twist in the opposite direction.

Quick Feet

This is a fun exercise, but it can be difficult to master. It uses all your muscles in a synchronous attempt to toss the ball from the floor.

Stand with the medicine ball on the floor between your feet with your knees bent. Then use your feet to "throw" the ball into your arm. To do this, you'll have to flex your knees and hips and power the ball up.

At first, you'll probably have to take a small bunny hop with your feet to get the ball in the air. Later you can bend your knees and actually throw the ball.

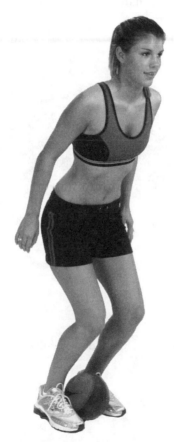

Quick Feet starting position.

Punch Ball

Punch Ball is a plyometric power-building exercise that shapes the muscles in your chest, back, and arms. You'll notice a firmer upper body and increased punching power after a few weeks of doing the Punch Ball.

Begin in a push-up position with both hands on the medicine ball. Push your arms off the ball and land in a push-up position with the ball an inch from your chest. Just as your hands hit the floor, hop back up to the starting position. Keep your back flat throughout the exercise.

Practice balancing with both hands on the ball before you attempt to push off. If this exercise is too difficult to perform from your feet, try it from your knees. If it's too difficult to "jump" with both hands simultaneously, perform the Punch Ball one hand at a time.

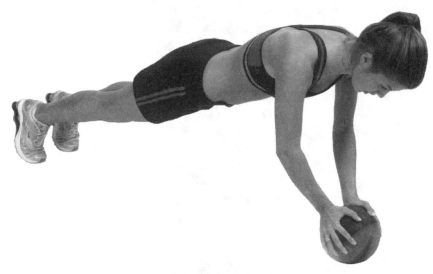

Punch Ball starting position.

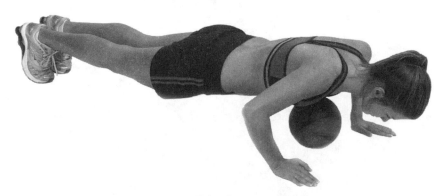

Punch Ball finishing position.

Chest Pass Punch

This exercise tones the upper body and works your balancing abilities. As you catch the ball, you must stabilize yourself so you don't fall off the stability ball.

Sit on the stability ball with your back straight, chest out, and stomach in. Have a partner perform the medicine ball chest pass with you.

Torso twist and overhead passes can also be done while sitting on the ball.

Make this exercise fun by playing hot-potato with the ball. As soon as it touches your hands, toss it back. Experiment with different foot positions to stimulate stabilizer muscles to maintain your balance.

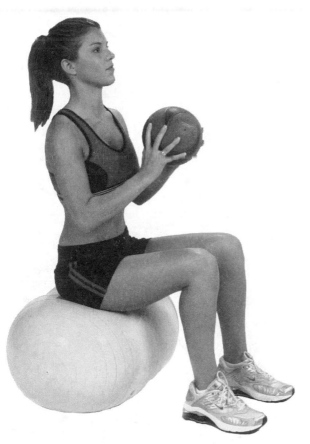

Chest Pass Punch starting position.

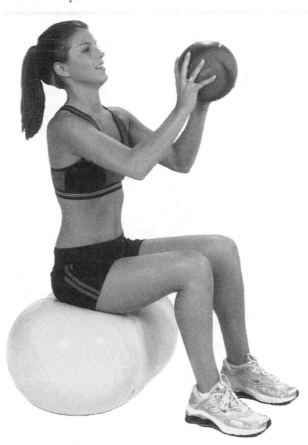

To challenge yourself as your balance improves, bring your feet closer together.

Crunch Pass Punch

Your abs, back, and arms get firm and toned by doing the Crunch Pass Punch. It's also a great way to develop sports-specific strengths.

Sit on a stability ball with your feet anchored firmly on the floor. Throw a medicine ball back and forth with a partner while performing sit-ups. Lean back just a few inches as soon as you catch the ball. Lean forward a few inches after the med ball leaves your hands.

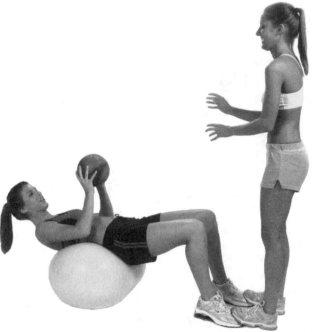

Starting position for Crunch Pass Punch.

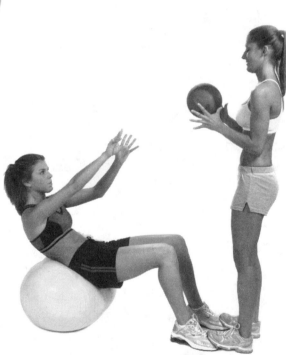

If you begin to tire, don't lean back as far during the crunch phase of the repetition.

The Least You Need to Know

◆ Tossing around a heavy ball is an effective way to build muscle strength and size.

◆ Simply play catch in the beginning. Don't try too hard, just have fun going through the motions.

◆ As you get stronger, increase the weight of the ball and challenge yourself by throwing faster. Be sure you maintain correct form throughout the range of motion.

◆ Hold the ball with both hands to minimize stress to ligaments and tendons. Be careful not to rear back and heave the ball with one hand.

◆ Find a like-minded partner to train with. If you don't have a partner, you can use a wall or rebounder, but it's a lot more fun to play catch with a friend.

◆ Basic throws and catches are all you need to get a firm and toned body. Trying to get too fancy can lead to injury.

In This Chapter

- ◆ Building better balance with a stability ball
- ◆ Starting out
- ◆ Upper body moves
- ◆ Lower body moves

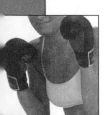
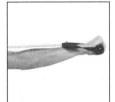
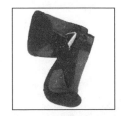
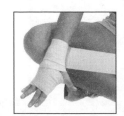
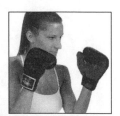
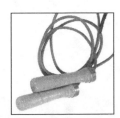

Chapter 8

Balancing on a Ball

Using an exercise or stability ball will help you develop better balance and stability—hence the name! Its round shape provides an unstable base from which to perform various exercises. As a result, stabilizer muscles strengthen and balance improves.

The stability ball also provides you with the chance to move through your exercises with a greater than normal range of motion.

When you do crunches from the floor, you lose about a 30-degree angle that you gain on the stability ball. This requires you to stretch muscles before you flex them. Stretching your muscles beyond their normal resting length on a stability ball gets more muscle fibers involved in your exercise. The more muscle fibers you use, the greater the toning effect.

Getting Your Balance

At first, brace the ball so it doesn't roll. Balancing on the ball is difficult enough without having to worry whether it's going to roll out from under you. Brace the ball against the wall or have a training partner hold onto it. You can also increase balance by deflating it slightly. Letting air out allows the bottom of the ball to flatten against the floor so that it's easier to maintain your balance.

Begin with easy exercises until you feel stable. As you get in better shape, you'll be amazed at how your stabilizer muscles improve your balance ability. Don't be tempted to stretch too far on the ball. Stretch just a little bit beyond the resting length of the muscle you are training. You should feel a light stretch.

Modify exercises to meet your needs. If an exercise is too difficult or doesn't fit your body correctly, change it. Just be sure to maintain appropriate posture and body alignment.

You should feel comfortable on the ball at all times. If your exercise feels uncomfortable, change it or have a spotter help you complete it properly. Rather than risk falling off the ball, modify the exercises to fit your needs and your ability level.

Knockout Punch

Some ball exercises can seem deceptively easy at first. Don't do too many repetitions the first day as your muscles will not forgive you the next day. Perform no more than 10 repetitions 3 days per week.

Now that you know how to use the ball and how to get your balance on it, let's do the moves!

Boxer's Crunch

The Boxer's Crunch is one of the best exercises you can do for your abdominal muscles, as it requires stretching the abs before flexing them. Doing crunches on the floor is not nearly as beneficial as performing them on a stability ball. On the floor, your abs aren't flexed through the full range of motion. When you lie back on the ball, you get an extra stretch on your abs that you don't get on the floor. This pre-stretch allows the entire abdominal area to work harder, and gives the following muscles a great workout:

◆ **The rectus abdominis.** This is the six pack that connects your ribcage to your pubis.

◆ **The external obliques.** These are the muscles on the sides of the stomach that make a "V" from your ribcage to your pubis.

◆ **The internal obliques.** These sit underneath your external obliques. They travel in the opposite direction, an inverted "V" connecting your ribs to your pubis.

◆ **The transverse abdominis.** This sits underneath all these muscles. It's a muscular corset that is activated every time you cough or sneeze.

All these muscles fire every time you throw a punch. You use them in lots of other activities, too, which is why it's so good to train them.

Sit on the top of the ball and get your balance. Your knees should be bent at 90 degrees and your thighs should be parallel to the floor. When you get your balance, move your feet forward until your middle back and shoulders are resting against the ball. You'll know you're in the right position when your hips are lower than your knees.

Bring your fists to your chin, as you would if you were in your boxer's stance. Now do a crunch, just as you would if you were on the floor. Contract your abs and exhale as you bring your ribs toward your knees. When you reach the top of the crunch, throw a jab and a cross. Perform 10 repetitions with correct form.

This exercise is excellent for torso strength, endurance, and recruiting stabilizer muscles. Because your lower back is comfortably contoured to the ball, you can perform more repetitions with less chance of lower back pain.

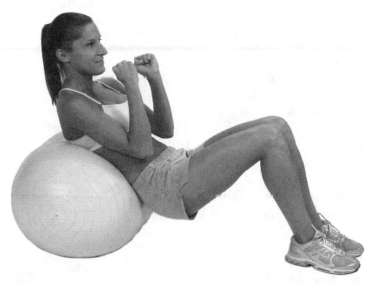

Be sure your lower back is resting against the ball. Keep your hands up and your elbows in.

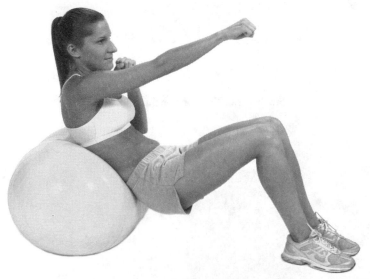

Execute your crunch and punch forward. The punches actually help you achieve the crunch as they pull you forward.

Punching Push-Up

Punching Push-Ups are an advanced form of regular push-ups from the floor. They work the chest, triceps, shoulders, and back.

Place the tops of your feet on the ball and your hands on the floor. Slowly lower your body to the floor, leading with your chest. Continue until your elbows are bent at a 90-degree angle. Pause for a second or two, and then push yourself up into the starting position. Keep your back straight when performing the push-ups—make sure you don't arch or sag. If you arch your back, you're putting pressure on your disks and spinal ligaments and may cause injury. Maintain a straight line from your shoulders through your elbows and down to your wrists. This keeps your shoulders, elbows, and wrists in proper alignment to prevent injury. This is also the power chain position you need for a strong punch.

Perform 10 repetitions using correct form. Add 2 repetitions a week as long as you can maintain correct form for each repetition until you can perform 20 reps.

If this exercise is too challenging, simply remain in the up position. Don't complete the move. As you gain strength and get a better feel for working on the ball, you'll be able to do the complete move.

 Corner Man

Punching Push-Ups can be tricky at first, especially if your balance on the ball isn't very good yet. Keep with it. Don't worry about how many repetitions you perform. One slow repetition with correct form is worth 10 repetitions of sloppy push-ups from the floor.

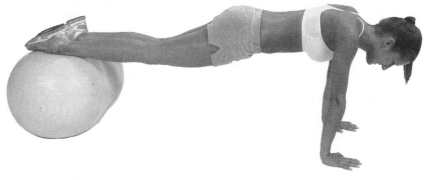

Starting position for Punching Push-Ups.

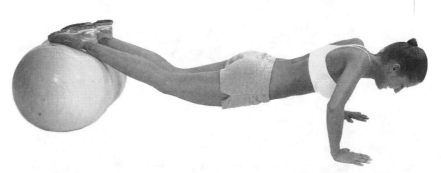

Keep your back as straight as possible when performing Punching Push-Ups. A little sagging is normal, but don't let your upper body sag more than this.

Boxer's Balance Push-Up

Boxer's Balance Push-Ups tone and strengthen most of the muscles in your upper body. They're also a fantastic workout for all the hard-to-get-to stabilizer muscles, which you'll realize immediately as your body shakes while attempting to maintain balance when doing these push-ups. When you can perform Boxer's Balance Push-Ups, doing regular push-ups will seem easy.

Place the balls of your feet on the floor and your hands on top of the ball with your back straight, chest out, stomach in, neck relaxed, shoulders, elbows, and wrists aligned.

Slowly lower your chest toward the ball until your elbows bend at a 90-degree angle. When you reach the bottom of the move (go no further than 90 degrees with your elbows), pause for a two-count. Maintain correct posture; breathe, balance, and focus on your core

strength. Exhale as you push yourself back up into your original position.

Perform 10 repetitions with correct form. Add 2 repetitions a week until you can perform 20 repetitions as long as you can maintain correct form for each repetition.

If this exercise is too difficult to attempt from your feet, try it from your knees. Secure the stability ball against a wall if you have difficulty keeping it still.

Corner Man

You might find that your entire body is shaking or quivering after you do balance pushups. This is actually a good thing, and nothing to be worried about. It means you've used all your muscles as you worked to maintain your balance.

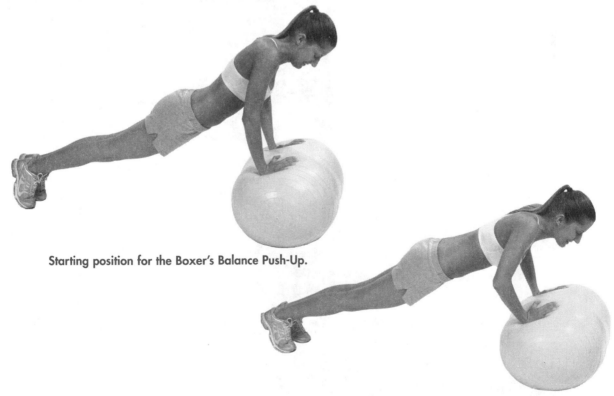

Starting position for the Boxer's Balance Push-Up.

Ending position for the Boxer's Balance Push-Up.

Kneeling Fighting Stance

This exercise is the beginner's version of the Standing Fighter's Stance, which is the next exercise in this chapter. This exercise is a full body workout. Although it might look easy, you'll use all the muscles in your abs and back to keep from falling off the ball.

Kneel on the stability ball with both knees. Keep your hands up in fighting position. You should immediately feel the core muscles of your abs and back trying to stabilize you as soon as you kneel on the ball.

Hold your position on the ball for as long as you can. Eventually work up to intervals of 30 seconds to 1 minute. Rest for a few seconds between 30-second intervals until you feel ready to tackle this awesome balancing task again. Eventually you'll be able to balance yourself for a full minute without help from your spotter.

When you achieve this level of fitness, perform the Kneeling Fighting Stance once or twice a week for 1 minute or so to stay in fighting shape. When this gets easy, try to hold the position with your eyes closed.

Corner Man

Although kneeling or standing on a stability ball might not seem like much of a workout, you'll use all your muscles to keep from falling off. At first, you might find yourself flapping your arms around madly as you try to stay balanced on the ball. If so, rest the ball against the wall or have a training partner spot you to prevent a fall.

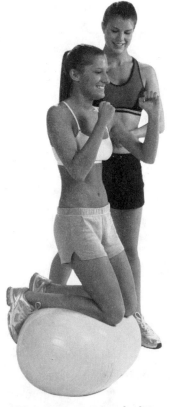

It's not as easy as it looks!

Standing Fighting Stance

When you've mastered the kneeling stance, you can work on this one. Or work on them both at the same time. This exercise trains every muscle in your body, from the small muscles in your feet to the larger muscles in your arms and shoulders. Mastering it without a spotter might never happen, as it's nearly impossible to do without assistance. People who try this exercise without a spotter end up spending more time falling than they do standing on the ball. It's great fun as long as you maintain your sense of humor.

If you don't have a spotter, place the ball in the center of a doorway. Stand on the stability ball with both feet as you use your arms to balance yourself on the sides of the doorway. At first, just lift your hands from the doorway for a second at a time and attempt to maintain your balance. After several months, try bringing your hands up into a fighting position—and keep them there.

Have a training partner spot you to prevent a fall. When this becomes easy, try to hold the position with your eyes closed. Hold the position for intervals of 30 seconds to 1 minute. Rest for a few seconds between intervals until your mind and body are ready to try again.

When you can stand on the ball for 1 minute without a spotter, pat yourself on the back. You're in the top 1 percent of the population with regard to balance training!

Be sure to practice the Standing Fighting Stance on the ball at least once a week to maintain your progress.

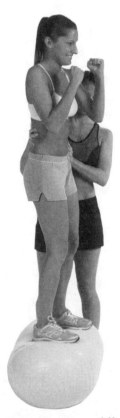

This exercise is 10 times more difficult than the Kneeling Fighting Stance. If necessary (and available), have two spotters help you keep balanced.

Boxer's Ball Lunge

The Boxer's Ball Lunge is a lower body toner and calorie burner. This exercise develops total body balance. The ball provides added resistance, and its size forces you into using many different muscles than if you were performing the lunge without equipment.

Stand tall, and hold the ball straight out from your chest with both hands. Be sure to keep your elbows soft to prevent strain. Keep your back straight, chest out, and abs tight. Step forward into a deep lunge and twist your torso to the side of the forward leg. Twist back as you step back into the starting position.

Alternate legs at first to give each leg a break between reps. When you've practiced this exercise for a few months, and you can do 10 reps on each leg with correct form without rest, try repeaters on the same leg for 10 reps. Then switch legs and do 10 reps with the other leg. When you don't allow rest between reps, your muscles work harder and tone up faster.

After several months of training, try performing alternating ball lunges across the length of the room and back.

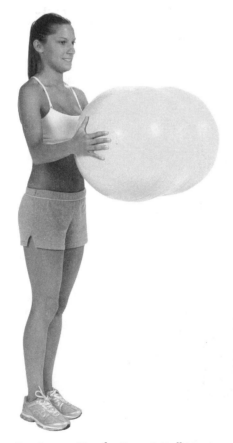

Starting position for Boxer's Ball Lunge.

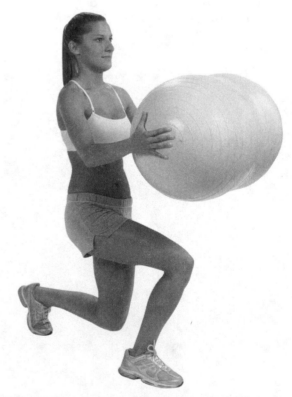

Ending position for Boxer's Ball Lunge. The farther you hold the ball away from your body, the more difficult the exercise.

Boxer's Ball Twist

Boxer's Ball Twists are a great way to isolate your upper body muscles. This exercise especially targets your side abs, or obliques, which are the muscles responsible for twisting your torso.

Position yourself on the ball as you did when doing Boxer's Crunches. Grasp a medicine ball with both hands. Keeping your elbows extended and arms perpendicular to your torso, rotate to either side. Maintain a relaxed neck

position. Be sure to keep your pelvis stable and just move your torso as you twist from side to side. This will focus the movement on your abs and keep them firing.

If you need to make this exercise easier, bend your elbows to 90 degrees. You can increase the difficulty by using a heavier medicine ball, increasing the speed of the movement, or by positioning yourself further back on the ball. Perform 10 repetitions with correct form.

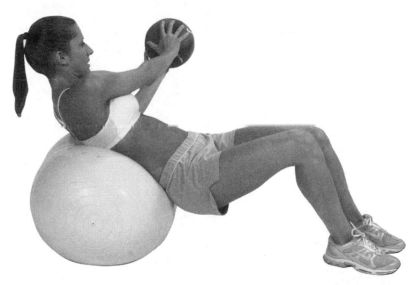

Focus on the muscles on the side of your abs rather than twisting from your hips.

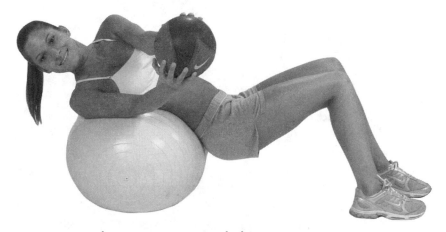

Focus the movement on your abs by just moving your torso.

Rocky Ball Roll

The Rocky Ball Roll is an upper body exercise that targets the abs and the back. It's performed at an angle that targets muscles you don't normally get the chance to train, which is one of the biggest benefits of this move.

Kneel and place the exercise ball directly in front of you. Clasp your hands and put them on top of the ball. Extend your body forward, moving in one line as much as possible, until your hips, shoulders, and elbows are fully extended. Hold for 1 second in the extended position before returning to the starting position. Return to the starting position by reversing the motion. Perform 10 repetitions with correct form.

At first, don't try to roll the ball too far. A few inches forward is fine for the first few weeks. Focus on keeping your back straight as much as possible—this will keep you in the proper position for this move and make your abs do the work instead of other body parts.

Knockout Punch

The Rocky Ball Roll is deceptively simple, but a real ab-killer if you do it right. If you can't maintain a straight back during this exercise, practice the push-up "up" position to strengthen your back muscles. Don't do more than a couple of reps at a time until you've been training for a few months. Later you can angle the ball off in different directions to target any area of your abs that you please.

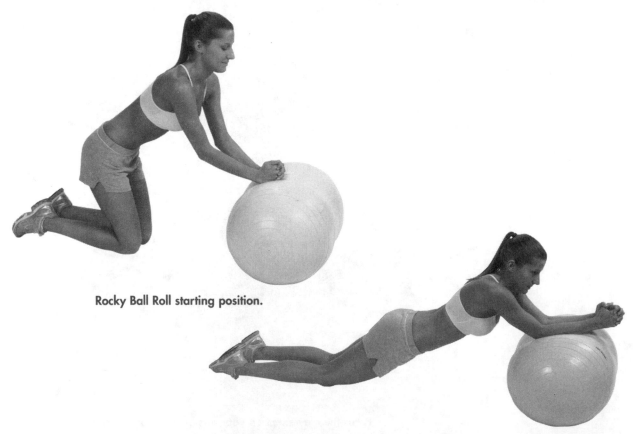

Rocky Ball Roll starting position.

Rocky Ball Roll ending position. At first, don't try to roll the ball too far.

Boxer's Leg Sweep

Leg sweeps on the ball are a higher intensity form of the same movement done on the floor. On the floor, leg sweeps are mostly an abs exercise. Done on the ball, they're a high intensity, full body workout. Your arms stabilize your body and your body stabilizes your legs. If you want ripped, toned abs, this exercise will get you there.

Place your ball a few feet in front of a chair. Lie face up on the ball, with your thighs parallel to the floor and your feet firmly planted under your knees. When you have your balance, flex your hips 90 degrees and raise your legs up in the air. Keep them straight and together, don't lock your knees. The top of the ball should be just under your lower back. Grab the chair that's behind you for support.

Starting with your feet pointing up at the ceiling, lower them to the right side until they're parallel to the floor. Return to center, and repeat on the left side. Your legs should look as if they were a piece of grass or wheat blowing back and forth in the wind as you lower and raise your legs from side to side.

Move your legs side to side only a few inches at first. If necessary, have a spotter help balance your movement.

Don't let your shoulders turn toward the direction your legs are moving in. This will cause the muscles in the side of your stomach to stop firing. When the legs are completely to the left, your right shoulder should be down, and vice versa.

Try this exercise from the floor before you try it on a ball. If you experience any back pain, try a different exercise such as ball twists.

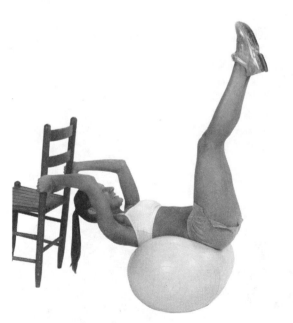

Starting position for Boxer's Leg Sweeps on the ball.

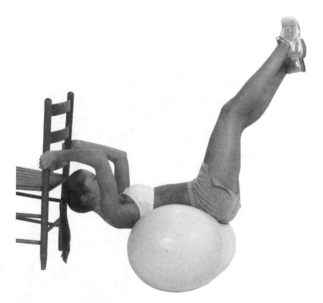

Ending position for Boxer's Leg Sweeps on the ball.

Fighting Position Roll

Similar to the Rocky Ball Roll—which works your upper body—except the Fighting Position Roll trains your entire body.

Kneel on the floor and place your forearms on the ball, making sure your hips and arms form a 90-degree angle. From this starting position, roll the ball forward as you extend your arms and legs simultaneously. Contract your abdominals to help support your lower back, which should not be strained. Roll as far forward as possible without dropping your shoulders or rounding your back. Do 10 repetitions.

To increase the difficulty of this exercise, hold the extended position for a second, and then return to the starting position.

At the completion of the Fighting Position Roll, your body should form a straight line with all your muscles firm and tight.

If this exercise is too challenging, remain on your knees throughout the exercise.

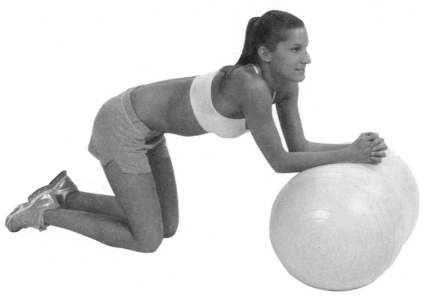

Starting position for the Fighting Position Roll.

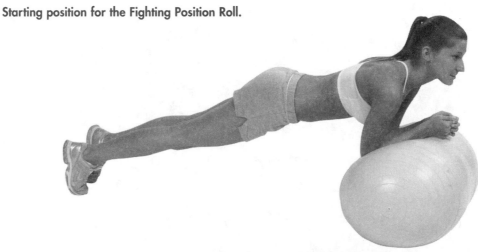

Ending position for the Fighting Position Roll.

The Least You Need to Know

◆ Using an exercise or stability ball will help you develop better balance and stability.

◆ When you're starting out, brace the ball against the wall or have your partner hold onto it. You can also take some air out of the ball for increased balance.

◆ Don't be tempted to stretch too far on the ball. Stretch just a little bit beyond the resting length of the muscle you're training.

◆ If an exercise is too difficult or doesn't fit your body correctly, it's okay to modify it to meet your needs. Just be sure to maintain correct posture and body alignment.

◆ You should feel comfortable on the ball at all times. If your exercise feels uncomfortable, change it or have a spotter help you complete it properly.

In This Chapter

- ◆ Powering up with free weights
- ◆ The benefits of weight training
- ◆ Choosing the right weights
- ◆ Best upper body routines

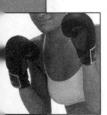
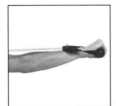
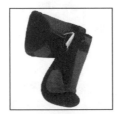
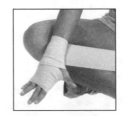
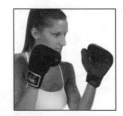
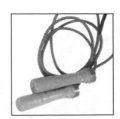

Chapter 9

Hitting the Weights

Strong athletes are better athletes, and lifting weights will make you both. When it comes to fitness boxing, strength training will also increase your explosive power and short-term endurance, both key factors for performing a boxer's moves with correct form.

This chapter focuses on weight training for the upper body. For lower body moves, turn to Chapter 3.

Why Weight Training Is Important

Weight training is great for gaining strength, but the benefits go way beyond this. Of everything you can do to stay fit, resistance training is your secret weapon for total fitness. Here's why: muscle fuels your metabolism. As you age, your body loses about six pounds of muscle per decade. The less muscle you have, the fewer calories you burn. If you continue eating the way you did when you had more muscle, you'll gain fat.

On the flip side, for every pound of muscle you add to your frame, you'll have to consume an extra 50 calories a day to support it. Putting this another way, you can eat an extra 50 calories a day without gaining fat. (Don't worry about the scale, by the way. If you're losing inches, gaining strength, and your energy levels are up, you're doing everything right.)

Resistance training also increases your bone density and decreases the chances of developing osteoporosis as you age. You don't necessarily have to build muscle for this; simply toning what you already have also works.

Maintaining muscle also increases the level of good HDL cholesterol in your body, improves your cardiovascular system, and helps prevent type II diabetes by using more oxygen and taking up extra blood sugar.

Fitness boxing stresses muscles at high intensities for short periods of time. Weight training increases your endurance and makes you less prone to fatigue when you're doing your routines. Some people worry that adding muscle will slow them down, but it won't. In fact, it makes you faster and more powerful.

Finally, weight training delivers quick results. After eight weeks of strength training, you'll notice improvement in your cardiovascular fitness, muscular strength and endurance, body composition, and flexibility.

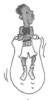

Sweet Science

Resistance training is the answer to a strong, sleek body. Although you can't spot-reduce fat, training with dumbbells can sculpt and shape your body.

Many women avoid weight training or do it only minimally for various reasons, but neither approach is a good idea. Done correctly, training with weights won't make you tight, sore, or cause you to tire out faster. In fact, these are all indications of overtraining or lifting incorrectly and should be avoided. Some muscle soreness is to be expected if you're new to lifting weights or haven't done it in a while. But any soreness you feel should be minimal and fleeting.

Weighting Up

It's easiest to do free weight workouts in a gym where you have free access to every size of weight imaginable. That said, you don't need a gym to do the workouts in this chapter. But you will need some free weights, and you'll need the right weights to meet your needs.

In general, you can lift heavy or light weights, depending on your goals. If you want to gain strength, lift heavy. If you're new to weight training, choose weights that you can easily lift 12 times using correct form. When you're new, it's important to learn which muscles should be doing the work. The combination of fairly light weights and good form will help you get a feel for using the correct muscles to lift and lower the weight.

Been lifting for a while? Challenge yourself to lift a weight that's heavy enough to become challenging as you approach your tenth repetition, again while maintaining correct form throughout the movement.

A workout pro? Choose weights that are heavy enough that you can barely finish your tenth repetition. Choose a weight that will only let you complete six to eight reps, max. Using heavy weights forces your muscles to adapt by getting stronger. Maintain correct form and use a spotter if necessary.

If your goal is muscular endurance, choose weights that allow you to complete 10 to 12 reps. Training lighter and longer will tone more than build, and will improve your endurance.

Knockout Punch

Use a steady, balanced cadence in lifting weights. Many times beginners use momentum rather than strength when lifting weights. Not only does this use muscles that are not supposed to be involved in the lift, it's also a surefire way to get injured.

You might also find the following equipment beneficial, but not a necessity:

◆ **Weight bench.** This piece of equipment facilitates better range of motion on things such as flyes and chest presses. A picnic bench or a balance ball are good substitutes. Do these moves on a balance ball, and you'll work your core, too.

◆ **Gloves.** Weight-lifting gloves can protect your hands when lifting heavy weights. Buy them fairly tight—you don't want them moving around when you're lifting.

Don't buy a weight-lifting belt. Instead of protecting the muscles in your back, they can actually cause injury by hampering development of the abdominal muscles. When you try to lift something—maybe your child off the floor or a piece of furniture—and you're not wearing the belt, your core muscles won't fire correctly because they're accustomed to being braced by a belt, which leads to the potential for injury. Instead, develop a muscular core to connect your upper and lower body.

Weight-Lifting Tips

There's definitely a right way and a wrong way to weight train. Adhere to these tips, and you'll be on your way to success:

◆ Maintain correct form throughout the movement. Don't arch your back too much and keep a neutral spine. Keep your shoulder blades back, your chest out, and your stomach in.

◆ Concentrate on moving the weight slowly through a full range of motion.

◆ Use steady and controlled movements. Count three beats up and three beats down. Never jerk or bounce the weights up and down.

◆ Breathe normally unless you're lifting heavy weights. If you're having difficulty performing the tenth rep with correct form, exhale on the exertion phase.

◆ Keep momentum out of the movement. Concentrate on keeping the muscles that you're training involved. Slow down so more muscle fibers are involved in each repetition.

◆ Don't lock your joints on any lift. Doing so can cause injury and diminish the benefit of the lift.

◆ Relax muscle groups that aren't part of the move.

◆ Vary the weight that you use so that you train both your fast- and slow-twitch muscle fibers.

◆ Be sure to eat right to fuel your workout.

Finally, never sacrifice good form for the amount of weight you're attempting to lift. Lifting weights correctly never injured anyone. Problems arise when enthusiastic lifters try to lift, push, or pull too much weight too soon. How much weight you lift isn't important. How you lift the weight is. Proper form is essential.

Best Free-Weight Workouts

The free-weight workouts in this chapter are safe and user-friendly. You can work any muscle group at any angle with them. Plus, they allow you to work out at any resistance and move at your own speed.

To learn the exercises and get your body accustomed to the resistance, do a full-body workout every other day for one month. Do one set of 10 repetitions for each muscle group at a weight that you can comfortably handle for all 10 repetitions.

Adding Intensity

After a month of training you can begin to add intensity to your workouts. This means training each muscle group only twice a week, but training your muscles using more weight. The harder you work your muscles, the more rest time they require to recover. Space your workouts as far apart as possible. For example a Monday and Thursday routine would be optimal. This allows for several rest days between each workout.

Each workout here is based on the overload principle, which calls for gradually increasing intensity to improve. Gradual is the operative word here. Whenever you can perform 10 reps with perfect form and with relative ease, add a little bit of weight.

Adding Weight

Add weight in the lightest increments available. For example, increase weight in 1-pound plates if you have them. If 2.5 pound plates are the lightest that you have, use them. Just be careful not to strain with the additional weight. Always maintain correct form, focus on the muscle group you're training, and be satisfied with a five to eight repetition range until your muscles adapt to the extra poundage, and you finally reach your goal of 10 reps.

When you first add weight, you might only be able to perform five to eight reps. That's okay. Continue to maintain your form and after a few weeks you'll increase your reps until you can perform 10. Continue this cycle and your muscles will become firm, tight, and strong.

Keep a record of your performance by keeping track of how much weight you use for each exercise. Objectively measure your day-to-day efforts by noting how much weight you were able to lift for 10 repetitions. This makes you accountable to your performance goals, which is important for your success.

Be sure to allow time for your muscles to recover after your workouts. Your muscles grow stronger and firmer when they're resting. Less is best when it comes to weight training. It's far better to train each muscle group twice a week rather than overtraining your body with an every day routine. In fact, if a muscle group is still sore from a previous session, don't train it. Your muscle is telling you that it hasn't fully recovered. If you "work through" the soreness, you'll continue to break down muscle. Without adequate recovery, your muscle cannot grow firm and strong.

> **Knockout Punch**
>
> More is not better with regard to your dumbbell training. Overuse injuries are common in those who are overzealous. Train each muscle group no more than twice a week.

Flye

A lot of the power in your hook comes from the pectoral muscles in your chest. To firm them up and make them look their best, there is no better exercise than Flyes. Here's how to do them.

Choose the weights you want to use, then lie down on your back. Extend your arms straight to the sides, at chest level, until they're almost locked, then raise them over your chest so that your hands almost meet at your center line.

Use enough weight to provide tension so you can keep the dumbbells moving smoothly and evenly. Keep your elbows bent at 90 degrees through the full range of motion just as if you

were throwing a hook. Feel your chest working. Keep your back straight. To prevent shoulder problems, don't let your elbows descend below parallel.

 ### Corner Man

Perform each exercise through the full range of motion, which is about 1.2 times the resting length of the muscle. Taking your muscle through a full range of motion means that you allow the muscle to fully stretch before you flex it. Rather than performing partial reps that don't engage your muscles fully, allow your muscles to lengthen before you contract them.

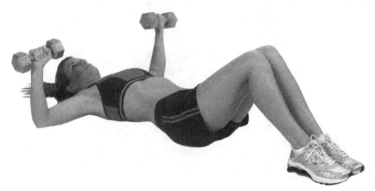

Keep your neck relaxed and your lower back flat.

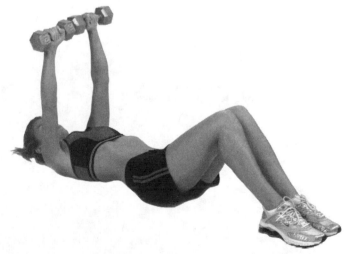

As you finish the move, be sure to keep your elbows unlocked.

Lateral Raise

Lateral Raises work the muscles on the outside of your shoulders and help you attain a V-shaped physique. Do enough of these, and you'll never have to wear shoulder pads again.

Stand with a dumbbell in each hand. Your feet should be approximately shoulder-width apart. Lead with your elbows and slowly raise your arms to the side, parallel to the floor.

Feel the weights in your hands as you raise and lower them—the dumbbells should provide tension in both directions.

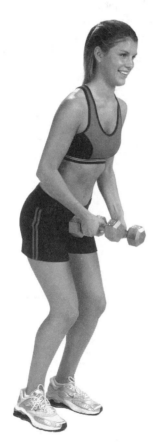

Lift your elbows no higher than parallel to your shoulders.

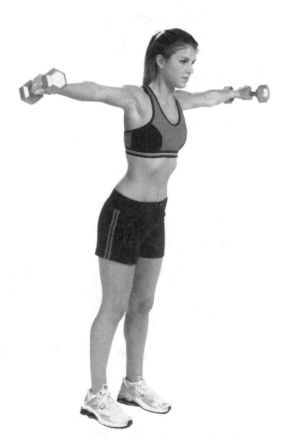

Move slowly on the way down to get the full benefits.

Front Raise

Front Raises round out your shoulders. Do them each time you do lateral raises to create symmetry in your shoulder muscles.

Grasp the dumbbells with your hands about shoulder-width apart and your palms facing downward in front of your thighs. Keep your knees and elbows slightly bent, and slowly raise the handles toward your head.

Pause when your arms are parallel to the floor, and then slowly lower them back toward

your thighs. Keep your thumbs up to protect your shoulders.

Corner Man

On lateral, front, and rear deltoid raises there is no reason to risk shoulder impingement by lifting the weights above shoulder level. You should always be able to see your hands with your peripheral vision.

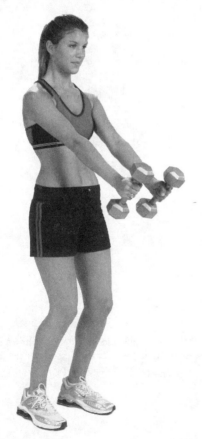

Be careful not to throw the weights into position. Move the dumbbells slowly both on the way up and on the way down.

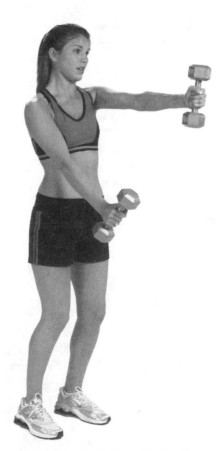

Raise the dumbbells no higher than parallel to your shoulders.

Shrug

Shrugs help build strength and definition in the trapezius (traps), or upper shoulder muscles.

Grab the dumbbells with an overhand grip, palms down, your hands shoulder-width apart, and your arms down to your sides. Keep your elbows soft as you shrug your shoulders toward your ears with the dumbbell providing resistance in both directions. Bring your shoulders straight up toward your ears without a rolling motion.

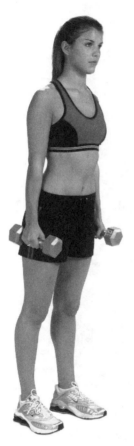

Be sure to begin with light weight on Shrugs so you don't injure your trapezius muscle.

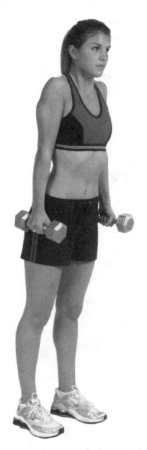

Resist the temptation to jerk the weight up into position. Move the weight 3 seconds up and 3 seconds down.

Back Attack

Imagine throwing a punch. Now visualize the muscles used to stop your punch and pull it back. This large back muscle is called your latissimus dorsi (lats). These muscles are a big part of fitness boxing, and they "V"-taper, which makes your waist appear smaller.

 # Bent Over Row

Grab a dumbbell with your right hand. Lean forward, and put your left hand on your left knee to brace your upper body. Extend your right arm straight down until you feel a pulling sensation in your back. Use the area you feel this sensation in to power up the weight until it reaches your ribcage. Do a full set of reps on this side, then reverse and work the other side. Keep your back as flat as possible; resist the temptation to hunch forward.

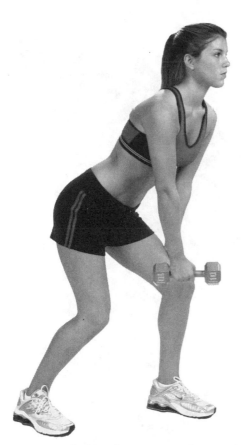

Hinge at the hips, keep your neck neutral, and bend your knees.

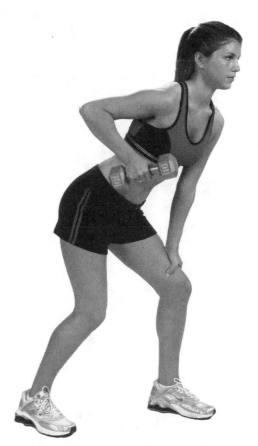

Keep your torso almost parallel to the floor as you pull the weight up toward your chest. Keep your elbow close against your body.

Push Your Punch

The triceps muscle in the back of your arm is responsible for adding the "pop" at the end of your punch. It is horseshoe shaped, and when it's firmed up it adds power to your physique.

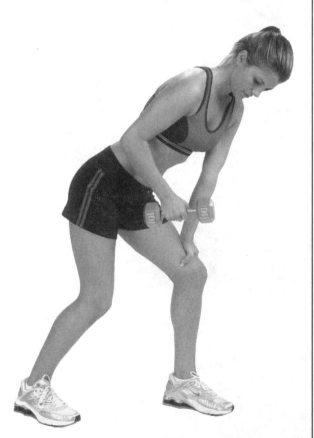

Be sure to hinge at the hip to protect your lower back.

Triceps Kickback

From standing position, grasp a dumbbell in your right hand. Bend forward from the hips and support your body with your left hand on your left leg. Bend your right arm at a 90-degree angle, then extend your lower arm straight back until your elbow is almost locked. Hold for 1 second and then return to a 90-degree angle. Do a complete set of reps on this arm, then switch and repeat with your other arm.

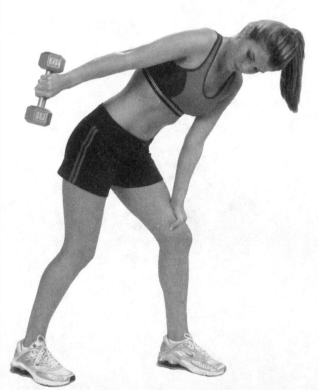

Begin with a very light weight and concentrate on your form.

Biceps Curl

The biceps play a big role in stopping and retracting your punch back to the fighting position. They're a big "show off" muscle, but they're also an important muscle group in fitness boxing.

You can do this one standing or sitting. From standing position, grip the dumbbell with your right hand and support your elbow with your left hand. This will isolate the movement and focus it where it should be. Lift and lower the weight through the full range of motion. At the peak of the contraction, go ahead and squeeze your biceps for a split second before allowing them to descend back to the original position. Don't lock your elbow when you move the weight down.

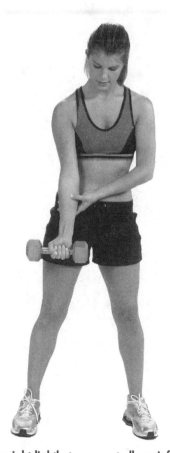

Grasp the weight lightly to prevent elbow inflammation.

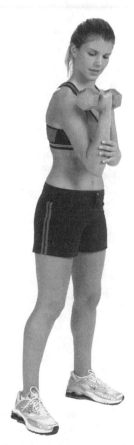

At the peak of the contraction, squeeze your biceps for a split second.

Reverse Curl

Reverse Curls train your biceps and forearms. If you don't have a lot of fat in these areas, they'll also give you a ripped, vascular look.

Grip the dumbbells at thigh level with an overhand grip. Your hands should be a little less than shoulder-width apart. Bring your arms up from the waist to shoulder level until your biceps touch your forearms. Lower the handles back down to your thighs using your elbows as the fulcrum.

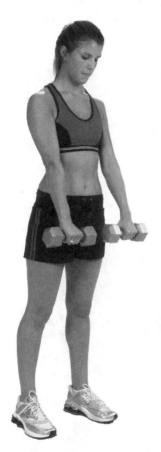

Do not swing the weights up. Move them slowly without using momentum.

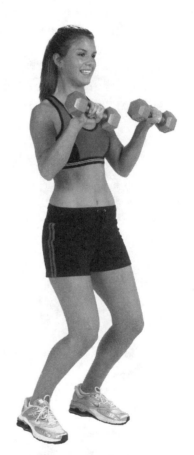

Keep your wrists neutral to prevent injury.

Pullover Stretch

Pullovers are great for working your chest and getting a good stretch at the same time.

Lie on your back and grasp a dumbbell with both hands. Extend your arms over your back, feeling the resistance of the dumbbell as you move. Return to the starting position, again feeling the stretch in your upper chest.

You should really feel your chest muscles working during this exercise. Concentrate on feeling your chest muscles contract every inch of the way through each repetition.

The Least You Need to Know

◆ Training with weights improves your outward appearance and has far-reaching effects on your fitness. Sculpt your body, improve your health, and enhance your punching performance.

◆ Strength training increases your explosive power and short-term endurance, both key factors for doing fitness boxing moves correctly.

◆ Never sacrifice form for weight. Lifting too much weight uses momentum, not strength, and makes you cheat on your form.

◆ Stop a movement immediately if you feel pain.

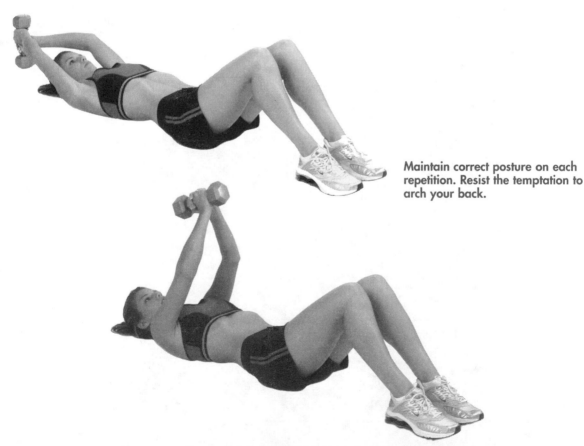

Maintain correct posture on each repetition. Resist the temptation to arch your back.

Keep your elbows slightly bent and your neck relaxed throughout the entire exercise.

In This Chapter

- ◆ Training together
- ◆ Feeling the flow
- ◆ Drills for balance and strength
- ◆ Manual resistance moves

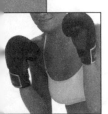 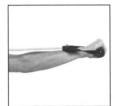 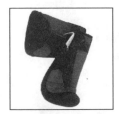 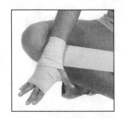 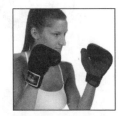 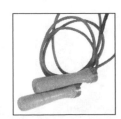

Chapter 10

Partner Exercises

Partner exercises can take your workouts to a new and very different level. Instead of depending solely on your own energy levels, you feel your partner's energy and move with it.

The moves in this chapter can help you and a training partner reach new levels of strength, muscular endurance, and balance. And they can be a lot of fun!

Wheelbarrow

The Wheelbarrow is a great exercise for firming and toning your arms, shoulders, chest, back, and legs. It also improves your balance and muscular endurance.

Lie flat on your stomach with your legs and feet together. Place your palms facing down underneath your shoulders. Now have your partner lift your feet off the floor while you keep your body and legs straight. She should only lift you a couple feet off the floor. Be sure your body is at no more than a 45-degree angle with the floor.

When that position feels comfortable, tell your partner you're ready. She'll then let go of one of your feet, which will require you to balance with one leg. Try to do it for 3 seconds. Then switch legs.

Now switch places with your partner and repeat the entire exercise. Be sure to communicate with your partner at all times.

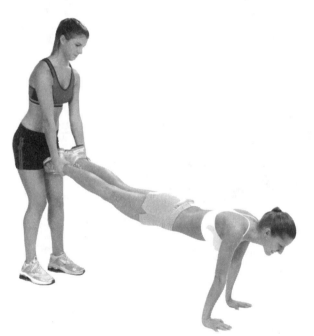

Keep your back and neck from sagging.

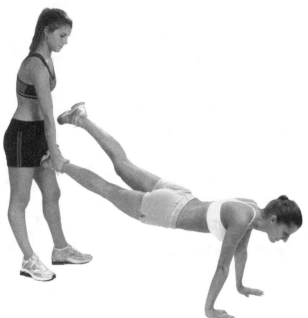

When your partner lets go of one leg, try to keep your back straight.

Reverse Wheelbarrow

The Reverse Wheelbarrow firms your buns, hamstrings, and lower back. It also engages your abs, which must stabilize your movement.

Lie flat on your back with your legs and feet together. Keep your arms at your sides with your palms facing down.

Have your partner lift your feet off the floor while you keep your body straight. Don't let her lift you more than a few feet off the floor. The angle of your body should be no greater than 45 degrees.

When you feel comfortable in this position, tell your partner to let go of one foot, requiring you to balance with one leg.

After 3 seconds, your partner should grab the extended leg and let go of the other one for 3 seconds.

Then switch places and repeat the entire exercise with your partner. Communicate with your partner throughout the entire exercise.

 Corner Man

Choose a training partner who has your best interests in mind. Help your partner achieve his or her fitness goals and your partner will encourage you to reach yours.

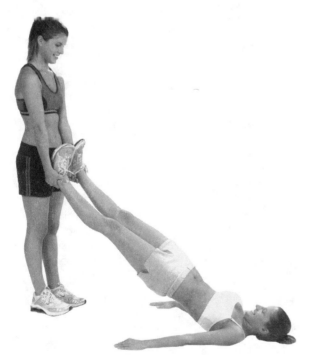

Maintain a straight back. The back of your shoulders, not your neck, should be on the floor.

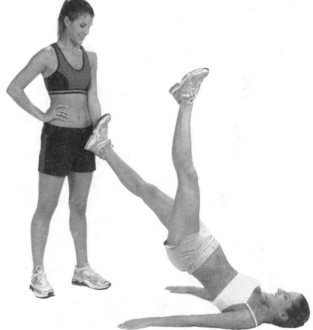

Keep your back from twisting sideways when your partner grabs and releases your legs.

Pushing Hands

This drill appears effortless but it works the core of your entire body the entire time you do it. Muscles in your abs and back must stabilize the blocking and attacking that you do with your arms. This burns calories and firms and tones your torso.

Stand facing your partner with your left foot forward, your elbows in, and your hands up. Your partner takes the same stance. Touch hands with your partner, then maintain light contact with your partner's hands, moving them in a circular motion.

When this circular motion becomes automatic, try to touch her body with one of your hands. Her response should be to deflect your hand while continuing the circular movement. Her response should be smooth and relaxed. Quick, flexing movements should be avoided.

Switch sides after 30 seconds and let your partner try to reach you. Deflect her strike with an effortless, relaxed circular block.

After 30 seconds, try to touch each other at the same time. Block each other's attempt without muscular effort.

Finally, close your eyes and continue blocking and attacking for another 30 seconds.

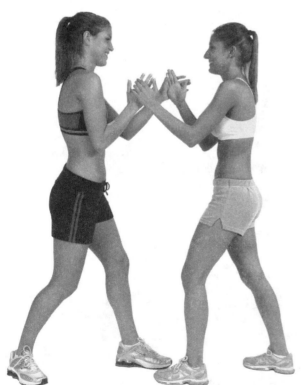

Maintain correct posture while you try to keep your arms relaxed. Begin all your movement from your abs.

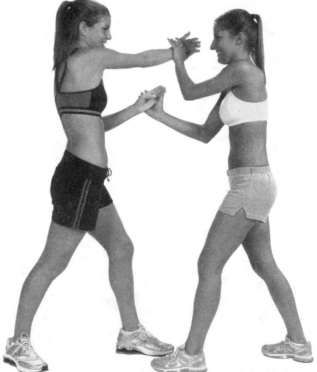

Keep your movements slow and smooth.

Balance Drill

This exercise is a full body muscle toner, from your lower legs to your upper shoulders. It burns a lot of calories but is so much fun that it doesn't feel like you're exercising.

Stand facing your partner in a fighting stance. Place your palms against your partner's palms. Attempt to push your partner off balance. Push and release. Try to make your partner move her feet to catch her balance.

When your partner pushes against you, you must push back. She is trying to do the same to you so you must keep a low center of gravity. To do this, keep your knees bent and your upper body relaxed.

Although this exercise might seem adversarial, try to feel the energy and muscular tension in your partner's body so you can short-circuit her attempt to break your balance. If you catch her at the right time, you can release your hands and she'll be thrown off balance.

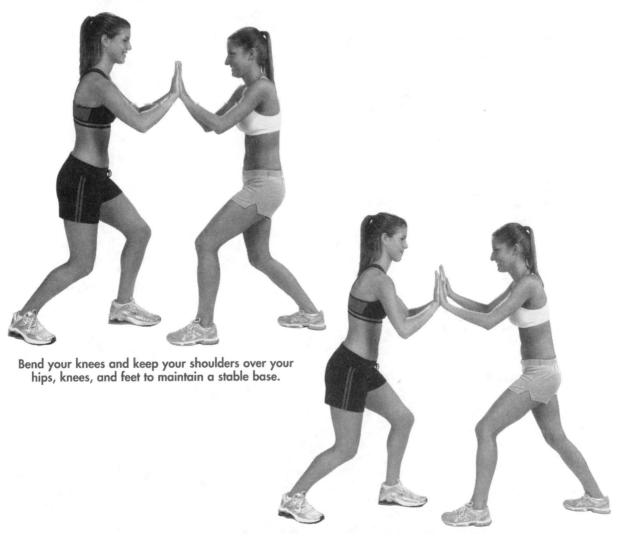

Bend your knees and keep your shoulders over your hips, knees, and feet to maintain a stable base.

Maintain contact with your partner's hands unless you pull away from her to throw her off balance.

Push-Up (Hand-to-Hand)

Partner Push-Ups firm and tone all the visible muscles in your body and some of the invisible ones, too. Your chest, back, shoulders, and arms do most of the work, but small stabilizer muscles are firing to keep you from losing your balance.

Lie down on your back with your arms up directly over your shoulders. Your partner places her hands against your hands as her feet straddle your feet.

When you're both in a square, comfortable position, begin to bend your arms into a push-up position. Maintain correct posture and try to move together, completing each Push-Up simultaneously. After you've performed 10 Push-Ups, switch places and repeat.

Although you may feel like a circus performer doing this move—and you're having a great deal of fun—be careful to keep your concentration so you don't lose your balance.

Knockout Punch

It's extremely important to maintain constant communication with your partner on all partner exercises. In many of these exercises, the training response you desire is in your partner's hands.

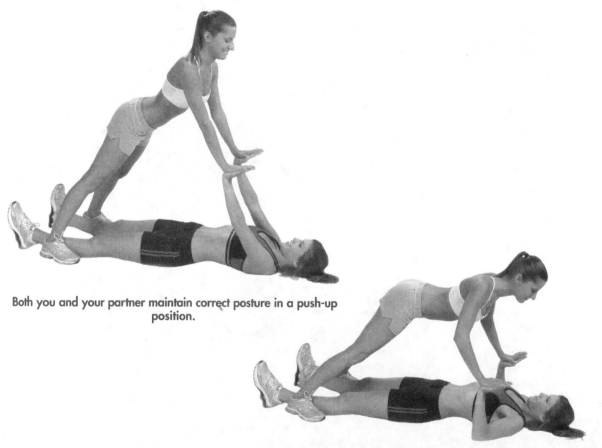

Both you and your partner maintain correct posture in a push-up position.

You don't have to bend your arms at a 90-degree angle unless you feel comfortable doing so. Even a slight elbow bend creates a useful training effect.

Manual Resistance

Manual resistance exercises allow both partners to receive a great upper body workout at the same time. When you push, your partner pulls and vice versa. These exercises are also a great way to isolate muscle groups and train them to reach their full potential with regard to strength, size, and tone.

Move very slowly through these exercises so that momentum isn't a factor. Three seconds up and three seconds down is a good tempo to maintain. Maintain perfect posture and move through a full range of motion on each exercise.

Place enough resistance against your partner so she's challenged for 10 repetitions. Exhale during the exertion phase of each repetition. Be sure to tell your partner if the resistance is too much, too little, or perfect.

 ## Biceps

Face your partner with your hands in fists. She has her palms down and you have your palms up. Both of you have your elbows bent at 90 degrees. As she presses down you press up. Move very slowly back and forth while you complete biceps curls and she completes triceps extensions.

Try to move through a full range of motion very slowly so you activate as many muscle fibers as possible. Consciously flex your biceps at the top of each repetition. Continue for 10 reps.

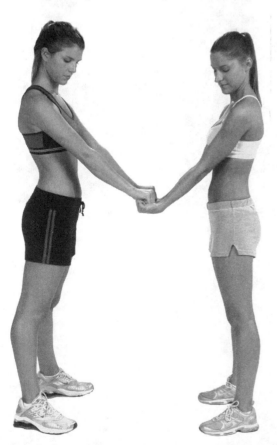

Keep your feet shoulder-width apart and bend your knees slightly. Your elbow is the fulcrum as your hands move from an extended arm position to a 45-degree angle at the top of the repetition.

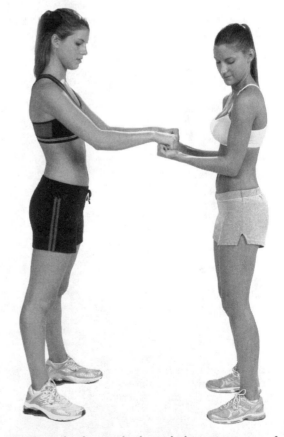

Keep your back straight through the entire range of motion. Use your biceps muscle to do the work instead of allowing your body to become involved.

Triceps

Repeat the biceps exercise but simply trade roles. This time you extend and your partner flexes. Begin with your elbow bent at a 90-degree angle with your palms facing down. Keep your elbows in close to your body and your back straight throughout the entire exercise. Your partner's palms are facing up and she provides resistance as you extend your elbows toward the floor. Exhale on the exertion and move slowly through each repetition. Continue for

10 reps. Be sure to tell your partner if she needs to provide more or less resistance.

 Corner Man

On all manual resistance exercises, provide enough resistance so that your partner is challenged on each repetition. If either of you breaks form, stop the exercise immediately.

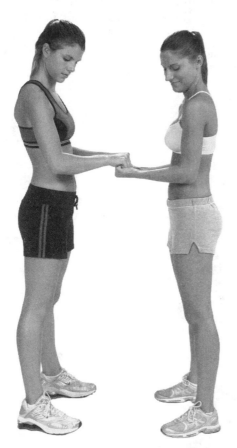

Keep the rest of your body out of this exercise by extending only at the elbows and keeping your back straight.

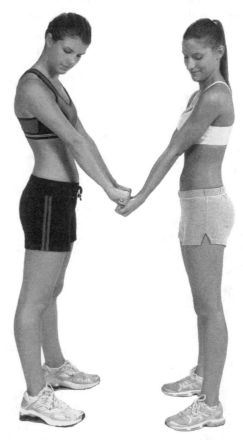

Press through each repetition with resistance in both the up and down direction to work all aspects of your triceps muscles.

Chest

Both of you are working your chests on this exercise. Face your partner and place your hands against her hands. As your partner extends her elbows, you provide resistance. Then you extend your elbows and your partner provides resistance. Move slowly and purposefully through a full range of motion focusing on the muscles in your chest throughout the exercise.

Keep your knees bent, back straight, and maintain correct posture throughout the exercise. Perform 10 reps.

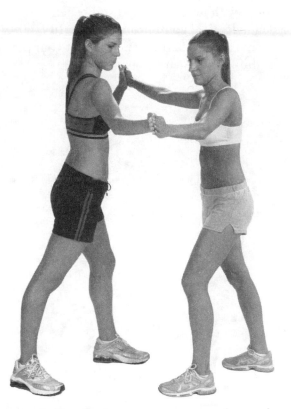

Instead of leaning into your partner, use the muscles in your chest as you press into your partner's hands.

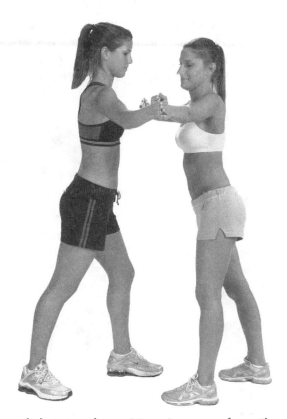

Exhale into each repetition using correct form. Three seconds out, three seconds back.

Body Work

Body work is a great way to firm your abs. It's fun and gives you the confidence to know that you can take a playful punch. Because there's no hard punching, it's a great body awareness exercise that teaches you to selectively contract specific muscles in your abdominal area.

Place a target pad over your abs. Your partner throws an easy punch that touches the target pad. Move the pad to your right obliques. Once again your partner lightly punches the pad. Move the pad to your left obliques. Your partner punches again. Each time your partner punches, contract the area of your abs where the punch lands.

Give your partner the pad and you throw the punches. While your partner is practicing contracting her abs, you're practicing correct form on your punches. You can do body work with or without contact and still benefit from your abdominal contraction. Throw 10 punches at your partner and then let your partner throw 10 punches your way.

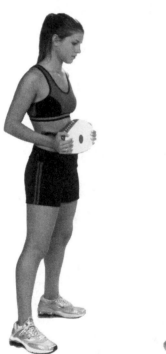 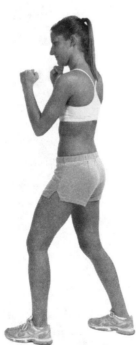

Stand facing your partner with a focus mitt placed against the front of your abs. Each time your partner touches the focus mitt with a punch, move it to a different location on the side of your abs.

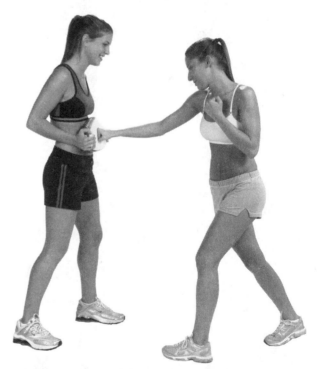

Tell your partner if she's pushing too easy or too hard. Exhale on each punch.

The Least You Need to Know

◆ Partner training is fun, but be sure to maintain your focus. It's easy to get a little distracted when performing some of these drills.

◆ Make your workout mutually beneficial by respecting your partner's wishes and intentions and by telling him or her what yours are.

◆ Always communicate with your partner, letting him or her know if you need more or less resistance.

◆ When doing manual resistance or body work, be sure to increase resistance incrementally rather than all at once.

◆ Never rush through these movements. Partner exercises are designed to improve your spirit of flow—feeling the energy of your partner and moving with it.

◆ Don't compete; do what you can do. Your partner may be bigger and stronger than you are. Do the best you can given your fitness level.

In This Part

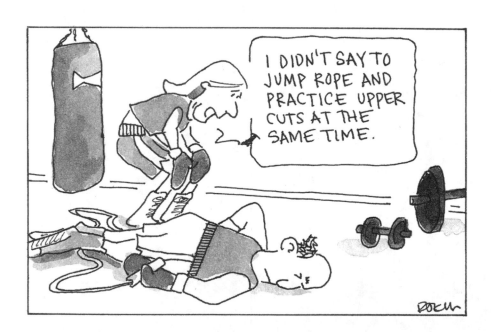

Becoming a Contender

By now you realize that boxing may not be as easy as it looks. A pro boxer makes all the punches and footwork look simple. Endless hours of practice make boxers appear effortless in the ring. The good news is that all your hours of practice will get you the toned and lean body you desire.

Part 3 shows you all the details you need to know, from the basic boxer's stance to the exquisite beauty of a well-executed punch. The "sweet science" of boxing is just that. From footwork drills to proper resistance training, you'll learn to move with a sense of grace and power. After learning all the fun and exciting exercises presented in Part 3, you'll never go back to a boring stationary bike or treadmill.

In This Chapter

◆ Standing—the right way

◆ Learning the basic boxer's stance

◆ Perfecting upper and lower body positions in the fighting stance

◆ Putting balance and gravity to work for you

◆ The correct way to breathe

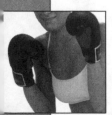 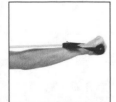 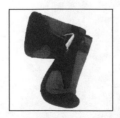 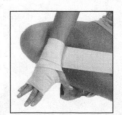 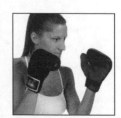 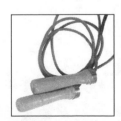

Chapter 11

Taking a Stand

We tend to take the way we stand—and, for that matter, the ability to stand—pretty much for granted as we go about our everyday lives. But in fitness boxing, the way you stand can make a big difference in the benefits you derive from your workouts.

In this chapter, you learn why standing the right way is so important to success in fitness boxing, and how it facilitates proper movement throughout fitness boxing workouts. Breathing correctly is also a big part of standing correctly, and about making your workouts the best they can be—which you'll learn more about here, too.

Separating Man from Animal

Our ability to stand upright is one of the things that separates us from the rest of the animal world. And although we tend to take this ability for granted, we really shouldn't. It takes an amazing combination of structure and musculature to be able to maintain an upright position. In some respects, it's really a marvel of engineering.

In fitness boxing, you won't spend a huge amount of your time standing still. But you will spend the majority of your time on your feet. What's more, you'll be moving your feet around a lot; in fact, for most of the time when you're working out. To do so, you need to be light on your feet and relaxed. If you're not, you'll tire out fast.

One of the keys to being light on your feet and relaxed is learning how to stand correctly (the other is breathing correctly, and we'll get to that later in this chapter). Doing so will make your fitness boxing routines as productive as they can be, which is why learning the mechanics of the boxer's stance is so important.

Sweet Science _____

Simply standing still burns a certain amount of calories as your muscles work to keep you erect. The way you stand when you're fitness boxing burns even more calories as you work to keep your abs tight, your back straight, and your arms lifted.

Basic Boxer's Stance

Fitness boxing uses a modified boxing stance. All movements in a fitness boxing program begin and end with this stance.

Learning how to do it correctly will help you stay fit, as just standing in the boxer's stance engages all your muscles. You're on the balls of your feet so your calves are flexed. Your knees and hips are flexed, which contracts the muscles in your thighs, hamstrings, and buns. Your arms are working hard to hold your hands up next to your face.

Learning how to do it correctly is also good for your back, which takes a lot of abuse during the normal course of things. Standing incorrectly can put an immense amount of pressure on your spinal disks and ligaments. Standing correctly alleviates this pressure and goes a long way toward making your workouts injury-free.

We start with the basic position for the entire body. Then we focus in more specifically on how to position your upper and lower body in the fighting stance, which prepares you to make your moves.

Corner Man _____

Practice the positions in this chapter—if possible, in front of a full-length mirror—as often as you can. Doing so will help you perfect them faster.

 Basic Body Position

Face forward and stand naturally, with your feet together (not tightly together, just next to each other) and your arms down at your sides (again, not tightly, just hanging there). Your hips and shoulders should be in alignment. Don't slump; there should be a natural curve in your back, but your pelvis and hips shouldn't be too far forward or back. If you're standing correctly, you should be able to just see the tips of your toes when you look down.

Imagine a vertical line running from the top of your head to the space between your feet. It should be straight. Keep your head level, with your chin relaxed and your eyes facing forward.

Without changing your basic alignment, move your feet comfortably apart. For most people, this is shoulder width or just slightly more or less than shoulder width. Distribute your weight evenly, and keep your knees soft (slightly bent). Keep most of your weight on the balls of your feet.

This is the posture you want to maintain whether you're moving forward, backward, or side to side.

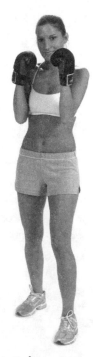

Basic boxer's stance.

Upper Body Position

To get your upper body into fighting position, first make your hands into fists, with the thumbs outside of your fingers, overlapping the index and middle fingers, and bringing your hands up to approximately chin level. Although your hands are in fists, you're not squeezing or clenching. Keep your elbows tucked in close to your ribs. Continue to keep your back straight and your upper body relaxed. Tuck your chin in slightly so it's protected by your left shoulder and right fist.

Now turn your body slightly sideways. If you're right handed, your left leg, hip, arm, and shoulder should be in front of your right (if you're left handed, obviously, you'll be positioned exactly opposite of this). Keep your entire body aligned with your leg and hip placement.

Your hands should be held high and your elbows tucked in to protect the body. Lastly, your chin should be "tucked" into your chest so that it's protected by your left shoulder and right fist. Although you're not going to fight anyone, this is the stance that will help maximize your workout.

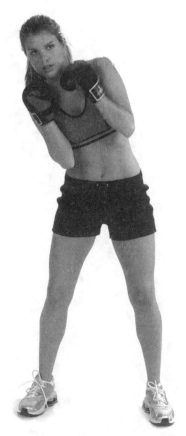

When you're positioned correctly, you'll be able to move your upper torso in any direction with ease.

Lower Body Position

To get your lower body into fighting position, simply flex your knees more to lower your center of gravity (you'll learn more about why this is important later in this chapter). Don't lock your knees—always keep them soft. Keep your weight mostly on the balls of your feet. This will help keep your feet light so you can move them at a moment's notice.

Boxers never square their hips to their opponents. Doing so places them off balance, doesn't let them pivot on the balls of their feet with their punches, and reduces their power and energy expenditure. Even if you never hit anything more than focus mitts or a heavy bag, you should follow this approach and keep your body angled toward your target as well. Doing so will not only help you move correctly, it will protect you from injury.

 Corner Man

Practice moving from a boxer's stance to a flexed knee position and back again until it feels natural.

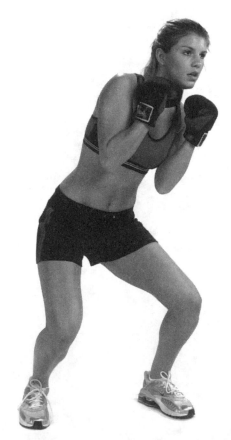

Stand with your feet shoulder-width apart and your weight equally distributed. Stand sideways to your imaginary opponent with your knees bent, elbows in, hands up, and chin down.

Working with Balance and Gravity

Both the boxer's and the fighting stance call for bending your knees and crouching quite a bit, which can be incredibly hard on your legs until you build strength and stamina. For this reason, it's tempting to just stand taller when you're working out, but this is a really bad idea for anything more than a few seconds or so. Here's why: balance and gravity are the two keys to really making the boxer's and fighting stances work the way they should. When you're crouched down, you're putting both factors to work for you. When you're standing up, you aren't.

The center of gravity of your body is at a point just below your belly button, or navel. Keeping your knees slightly bent and your shoulders over your hips will drop your center of gravity even lower—into your thighs—and help you use it to your best advantage—meaning that you'll stay better balanced.

To further maintain your balance, keep your feet positioned comfortably apart, and keep them in line with your hips and shoulders.

Knockout Punch

Keeping your feet too close together will narrow your base and upset your balance. So will crossing your feet when you do your moves. To maintain better balance, focus on keeping your feet comfortably apart, no matter what position they're in.

Developing a greater awareness of your center of gravity is essential for helping to build a stable base from which you can make all your moves without—you guessed it—losing your balance. Without this knowledge and awareness, it might be difficult for you to throw your punches at first, as you'll have a tendency to lose your balance and feel unstable.

If you have a workout partner, you can do a quick demonstration that will help you better understand how the body's center of gravity comes into play in fitness boxing. Have your partner stand normally, then grab her from behind and try to lift her up. Notice how heavy she feels, whether you can lift her or not.

Now ask her to relax her body. This will drop her center of gravity lower. Again try to lift her. If you couldn't lift her before, it should be even harder now. If you could lift her before, you probably won't be able to now.

The bottom line (sorry for the slight pun!) is this. The lower your stance, the stronger it is. That said, it isn't a good idea to make your stance *too* low, especially when you're first starting out. Doing so can tire out your legs too quickly and cause you to get sloppy with the rest of your body position.

Just Breathe

Breathing is simple. You do it all day and night, inhaling at least 15,000 times a day. But there's a right way and a wrong way to breathe, and most people do it the wrong way. Instead of filling their lungs fully, they breathe shallowly and only fill their lungs part of the way. This happens for a variety of reasons:

- **Age.** As we grow older, the muscles we use to breathe can become less efficient.
- **Posture.** Good posture is essential for breathing correctly.

◆ **Stress.** If you've ever had a panic attack before a big presentation, you've experienced the effects of stress on breathing—it results in shallow breathing and hyperventilation.

◆ **Illness and/or injury.** If you are ill or injured you might have a tendency to slump your shoulders and breathe from your upper chest instead of from your diaphragm.

Breathing incorrectly probably won't affect you much when you're just going about your daily routine, but it sure will when you start working out, and working out hard, as you will with fitness boxing. Jump rope for 3 minutes, and you'll quickly realize how breathing, or the lack thereof, can affect every cell in your body.

The lungs are designed to provide a sufficient and uninterrupted flow of oxygen to the blood when we inhale, and to eliminate carbon dioxide—the waste gas our bodies produce—when we exhale. If, for some reason, the lungs can't exhale enough carbon dioxide, it builds up in the body and poisons all the cells of the body.

Breathing correctly is essential to getting a better workout. You don't have to consciously remember to breathe—your brain stem automatically does this for you. But by focusing on how you breathe, you can learn how to do it better.

Understanding the Mechanics

When you breathe, your brain sends impulses down your spinal cord and to two nerves: the phrenic nerve, which controls your *diaphragm* (belly area); and the intercostal nerves, which control the *intercostal* muscles in your abdomen.

Clear as a Bell

The **diaphragm** is the muscular wall below the ribcage that separates the abdomen from the area around the lungs. **Intercostal** muscles are the muscles that are situated between the ribs.

When the diaphragm and the external intercostals contract, air is drawn into the body. The ribs move upward and outward, and the sternum moves upward and forward, which allows your chest, or thorax, to expand in three directions, and your lungs to expand.

Expiration, on the other hand, is done passively. All that happens is that the muscles used for inspiration relax.

The best breathing engages both the diaphragm and the abdominal muscles. Shallow or chest breathing, on the other hand, does not.

If your shoulders lift and/or your stomach doesn't move in and out when you breathe, you're a shallow breather.

Knockout Punch

Holding your stomach in might look good, but it's one of the worst things you can do for your body. Pulling in your stomach pushes the diaphragm up and hampers its natural movement when you breathe. Over time, this can actually minimize lung capacity.

Breathing from Your Belly

You want to learn how to breathe from your belly, which helps you get more air to your lungs during activity. Belly breathing also helps you relax.

The following exercise will help you learn how to breathe from your belly:

1. Lie on your back and place your hand or a book on your belly.

2. Take a breath, and watch your belly. Your hand or book should move out as you breathe in.

3. Breathe out. Your hand or book should move back down to the starting position.

This might take some time to get used to, especially if you've been a chest breather for some time, and especially if you're used to holding your stomach in. If it feels really uncomfortable, practice it at various times during the day. Just place your hand on your belly and breathe. Remember, your hand should move out with your belly.

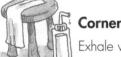

Corner Man

Exhale with every move you make to increase power. Exhaling increases your power, contracts your abs, and focuses your attention on your technique.

Focusing on your breathing, and allowing your breathing to occupy your thoughts, alters your attention and is also a great way to mentally prepare for your fitness boxing workout. Breathing correctly is also a great way to put more power in your punches, which you'll learn more about in Chapter 12.

The Least You Need to Know

- One of the keys to being light on your feet and relaxed is learning how to stand correctly. The proper stance is focused, yet relaxed.

- Always keep your body angled slightly to your target. Doing so will allow you to pivot on either foot when you throw your punches.

- Keep your hands up. It's a natural tendency to drop one when you're punching with the other one.

- Bend your knees to drop your center of gravity and build a stronger base for your moves.

- Breathe from your diaphragm. Don't hold your breath on punches. When in doubt, exhale with each punch.

In This Chapter

- ◆ The anatomy of a punch
- ◆ Lightning Left Jab
- ◆ Crossing power
- ◆ Hook 'em!
- ◆ Unleashing the uppercut

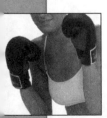
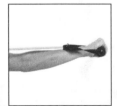
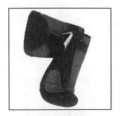
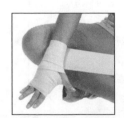
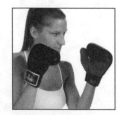
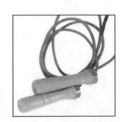

Chapter 12

Throwing Punches

You've learned the basics of the boxer's fighting stance. Now it's time to learn the correct way to punch. Although you may never step into a boxing ring or have to defend yourself in the street, it's important to learn the correct way to punch. Mastering these fundamentals is essential to building a boxer's body, which is your goal and the reason you're doing fitness boxing to begin with, right?

The jab, cross, hook, and uppercut are all fantastic for shaping the muscles of your upper body and building strength, and they're the foundation of your fitness boxing program. In this chapter, you learn the correct way to punch.

Fighting Position Review

All the punches in this chapter begin from the basic fighting position. Let's review what this is.

Face your opponent (imaginary or otherwise) slightly sideways. Your left foot and left hand should be forward, with your weight evenly balanced on both legs. Keep your chin tucked slightly into your chest—in other words, don't thrust it forward as this quickly leads to muscle fatigue.

Keep your hands next to your chin, with the left hand about 6 inches in front of the right. Even though you're not facing an opponent, boxing is all about protecting your face, which is why your hands are always up near your chin. Your thumbs should be next to your chin, facing each other and held about 6 inches apart. Try to resist the temptation to rotate your wrists too far inward, which will flatten your hands and move them out of punching position.

Keep your elbows tucked into your ribs. Look out over the knuckles of your left hand. This "targets" your punches, and keeps your body in proper alignment as you work. Keep your wrist in line with your forearm. Never fully extend your elbow—doing so puts strain on your shoulders and can cause injury to your shoulders and elbows. Keep your upper body focused, but relaxed.

Corner Man

Flying elbows—elbows that flap around like a bird—are a no-no both in the ring and in fitness boxing, as they result in sloppy, unfocused punches. Always keep your elbows down no matter what punches you're throwing. This keeps the muscles you're using to throw punches in proper alignment, and takes the pressure and strain off your shoulders.

All punches should be thrown actively—in other words, you're going to engage all your muscles when you do them. This means flexing the muscles in your lower and upper legs, which is where your punches start from (while it might look like punches are primarily upper body moves, they begin from the ground and work their way up your body), and pulling in your abs and keeping them tight. Then you'll use the muscles in your chest, shoulders, back, and arms to complete the punch. This creates a "power chain" through your body, starting from your foot and traveling through your leg, hip, abs, chest, and shoulder, and finishing in your arm through the fist.

This concept might be a little hard to grasp at first, but when you get the hang of it, you'll be able to feel your muscles working together as you deliver your punches.

Punches work your muscles in new ways and you're going to feel sore in unfamiliar and unexpected places until you build up your endurance. At first, throwing as few as 10 punches in a row might be all you can manage. But keep with it! In a few months you'll have increased your en-durance to the point where you can throw five times as many and be begging for more.

It's not essential to have the mechanics of the moves down perfectly, as striving for this can hang you up on the details and make you feel like you shouldn't do the moves at all. Safety is more important than perfection.

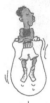

Sweet Science _____

Because all punches have a different purpose, and you throw all of them at different angles, you're performing four different full-body workouts when you do them.

Fist First

Although your goal isn't to be in a prizefight, it's still important to learn how to make a fist, as proper hand position is key to throwing punches correctly and protecting your knuckles when you're hitting a heavy bag or focus mitts.

Simply open your hand completely flat, then curl your fingers toward your palm. Roll them in tightly. Place your thumb across your index and middle fingers—not on top of your index finger. If you have long fingernails, you might find it difficult to make a tight fist. This isn't a huge issue if you're not going to hit anything, but if you are, you might want to consider cutting them down.

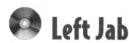 **Left Jab**

The Left Jab is the workhorse of the boxing world, and is the punch you'll throw more than any other. It's a fast punch, and it typically leads punching combinations.

Here are the points of the move:

1. Begin from the basic fighting position. Push off the ball of your right foot as you step forward with your left foot. Shift your weight to your front foot as you step forward.

2. Keeping your hands close to your chin, snap your left arm straight out. Your fist should travel straight to the target as your shoulder rotates slightly inward toward the centerline of your body. Remember to keep your wrist in line with your forearm— if a ruler was placed on the side of your arm, it would be flush with your wrist and forearm. Your fist also rotates inward as it nears the target so that the final position has your palm pointed toward the floor. Keep your elbows unlocked and your chin near your chest. Keep your right hand up in the guard position.

3. Pull your arm straight back to the starting position.

4. Immediately step back into your boxing stance. At this point, both hands should be in their original position.

Practice this punch slowly, using a one-two beat:

1. Snap your arm straight out from your chin.

2. Pull your arm straight back to the starting position.

Move slowly until you get the moves down correctly. Then throw a complete jab on one beat. Count "one," and throw out and back. When you have this down, try a series of eight jabs. Remember to step slightly forward as you throw, and return to the starting position when you complete the punch.

After you've trained for a few months, you should be able to snap the jab out quickly, with a fast delivery and recovery. If you're training with target mitts, you should hear a popping sound when your jabs hit them. In other words, the jab is like cracking a whip—as opposed to a cross, which is more like cracking a whip with a steam roller behind it, creating more of a thudding noise when thrown.

 Corner Man

If you're using a heavy bag in your workout, be careful not to push it when you throw a jab. The pushing motion slows your jab and you won't be able to throw as many. Instead, you should "pop" the bag. If you do this move correctly, you'll see the bag quiver when you hit it.

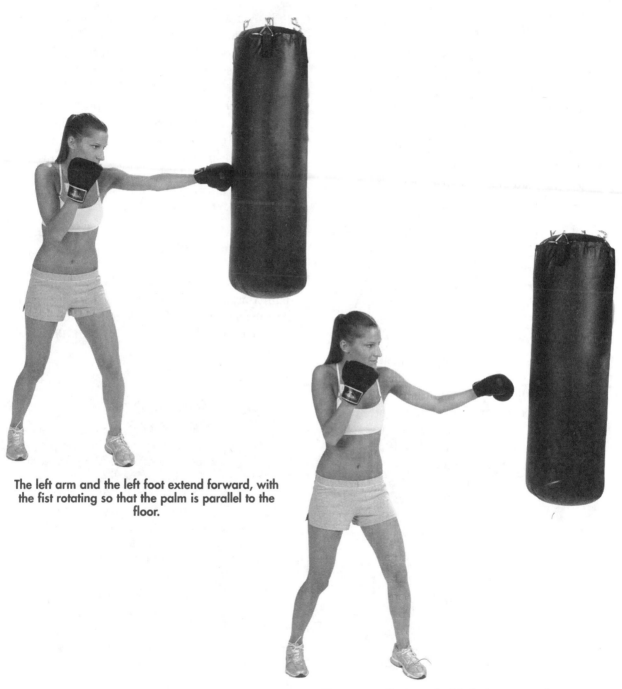

The left arm and the left foot extend forward, with the fist rotating so that the palm is parallel to the floor.

Keep your elbows tucked in between punches.

Right Cross

The Right Cross, sometimes called a straight right, is exactly what the name implies—a right-handed punch thrown across the body. It's typically thrown in combination with the Left Jab; first a jab, then a cross.

The cross, as well as the rest of the punches in this chapter, is a more powerful punch than the jab, and can be a little harder to learn.

Here's how to throw a Right Cross:

1. From the basic fighting position, pivot your right foot inward and slightly twist your right hip inward as well, away from your target. As you do, keep your right elbow down and close to your side. As always, your hands are up near your chin, protecting your face.

2. Using your right hand, throw the punch straight out from your chin. As you do, you should feel your right shoulder rotate forward and your left shoulder dip down slightly. Rotate your right palm toward the floor as you punch through. Be sure to keep your left hand near your chin, with your elbow near your side.

3. At the full extension of this punch, your leading foot (if you're right handed, your left foot) should be flat on the ground. You should be up on the toes of your right foot. Your right shoulder should be closer to your imaginary opponent than your left shoulder is. Your hips should be square to the target, and your chin should be down. The power of this punch is magnified by the rotation of the right foot, hip, and shoulder, while stepping forward with the left foot.

4. Pull your arm back, and return to the starting position.

Tighten your abdominal muscles to maintain your alignment. Keep your back straight. At the completion of the punch, exhale and contract your abs as hard as you can. Perform 10 reps with correct form.

Knockout Punch

When you throw a Right Cross, the muscles on both sides of your body need to contract and relax with perfect timing. Otherwise there won't be much power in the punch. As an example, if you extend your arm before you pivot your foot, you won't engage your back muscles in the punch. The result is an arm punch. There's little power in an arm punch, and it doesn't burn much fat or tone much muscle.

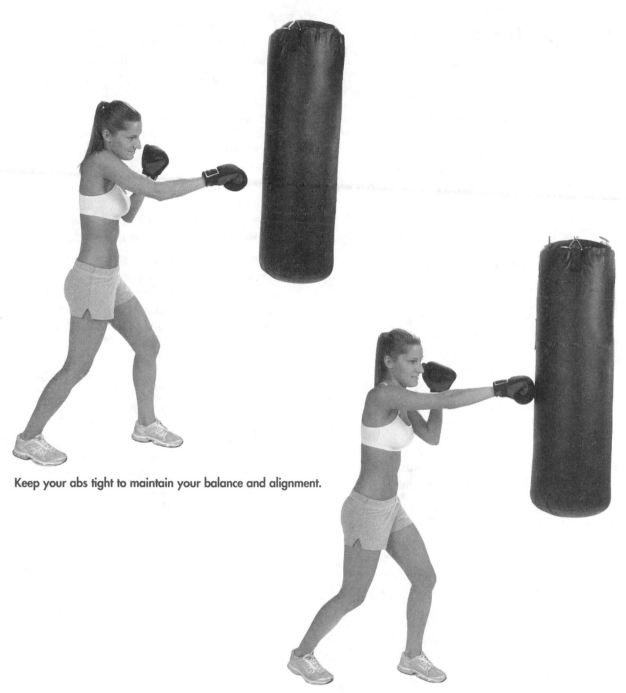

Keep your abs tight to maintain your balance and alignment.

Be sure to pivot your foot before you extend your arm.

Left Hook

Simply put, the Left Hook is a tough little punch to get down, as it can be difficult to coordinate, especially at first. In fact, it will probably drive you the craziest of all the punches. But don't let the difficulty of this punch deter you from learning it, and using it. Remember, all the punches use your muscles in different ways, so you don't want to miss out on the benefits of this punch.

Sweet Science

Want to see how the Left Hook works in the ring? Watch old fight films of ex-professional heavyweight champion Joe Frazier, and you'll see one of the best Left Hooks in boxing. Frazier threw Low Hooks, High Hooks, Lunging Hooks, and even Jumping Hooks.

Here's how to throw it:

1. From the basic fighting position, start with both fists in the same position as with a jab or cross.

2. Lift your left elbow parallel to the floor. Your left thumb should be up, and your knuckles should be pointing outward. Your arm should be in somewhat of a hook shape.

3. Pivot on the ball of your left foot so that the toes on that foot are pointed inward. Rotate your hips and shoulders from square to sideways, pointing to your imaginary opponent.

4. Keep your left elbow bent at a 90-degree angle. Sweep the punch across your body. Be sure to follow through. Keep your chin tucked throughout the punch as you would for all your punches.

When you complete this punch, your left hip should be pointed at your target.

The complexity of this move makes it essential to practice it in stages or segments at first. Eventually, you'll be able to combine each part into one flowing movement. To start, perform 10 reps with correct form.

Knockout Punch

Early in your training, be careful not to practice too many hooks consecutively. You'll feel more than a twinge on the obliques of the left side of your abs. Overtraining can make these muscles painful. Instead, practice all your punches at an easy pace.

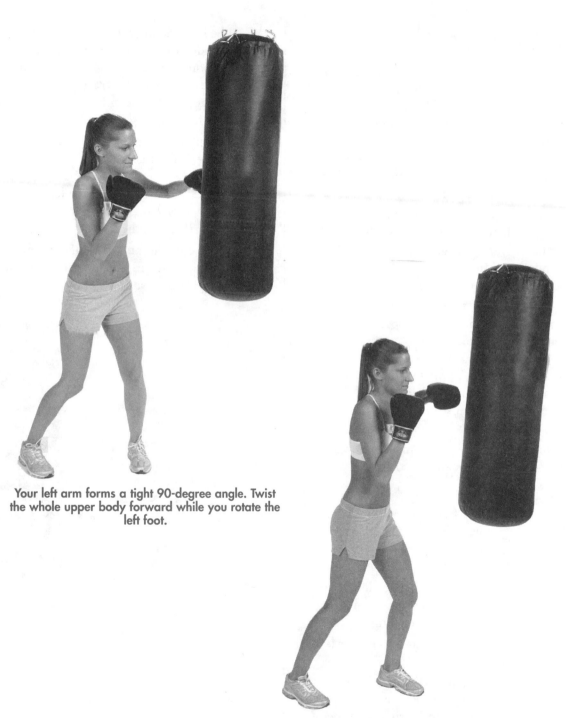

Your left arm forms a tight 90-degree angle. Twist the whole upper body forward while you rotate the left foot.

Extend the left arm to punch across the front of your body all the way through to the right side. Keep the right hand up in the defense position.

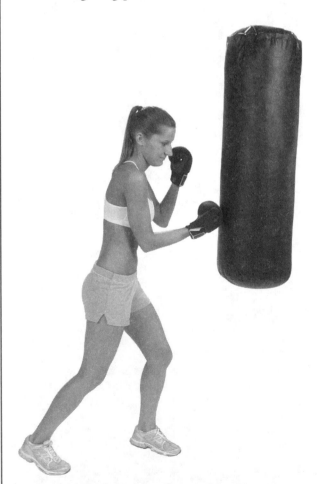 Uppercut

The uppercut is one of the most effective moves for toning many of the large muscle groups in your upper and lower body. You bend your knees for this more than for any other punch, and your upward movement is against gravity. After a few dozen uppercuts, you'll feel as if you have just completed "leg day" in the weight room.

You can throw your uppercut to head level or body level. You can throw this punch with either hand, but the Right Uppercut is a little more powerful. Just as in the Right Cross, you pivot your right foot, which lets you get more of your body weight into the punch.

The jab, cross, hook, and uppercut are all classic boxing punches. As such, there's no wind-up, no cocking your arm back before you throw any of them. Throwing your punch without cocking your arm back also burns significant calories because you keep your hands up and use your body to create power.

As mentioned, the power from the uppercut comes from your legs and torso. Here's how to throw it:

1. From the basic fighting position, with your hips squared to your imaginary opponent, dip your left shoulder so that your left elbow brushes your left hip.

2. At the same time, rotate your left fist so your palm faces the ceiling. Keep your elbow bent at a 90-degree angle.

3. Bend your left knee and rotate your left shoulder into a crouching position.

4. Drive off the ball of your left foot as you begin to rotate your hips toward your imaginary opponent. During the process, your elbow should be bent at a right angle during both the delivery and the follow through.

5. The left side of your back and your left shoulder will follow through with the rotation of your hips. Resist the temptation to extend and retract your arm. Instead, uncoil the entire left side of your body like a spring.

6. As you deliver the punch, your body weight will transfer to the ball of your left foot while you maintain a bent elbow. Explode the punch with the left side of your body as the punch is delivered with a bent arm at a right angle.

7. At the completion of the punch, rotate your hips back to your original side facing the fighting position.

Use your body to throw the punch, not just your arm. Begin by bending your knees and finishing with a follow-through of your arm.

Now try a Right Uppercut. Bend your right knee and lower your right shoulder into a crouching position. Drive off the ball of your right foot as you begin to rotate your hips toward your imaginary opponent. During this process, your elbow should be bent at a right angle both during delivery and follow-through. The right arm always stays close to the body and moves upward in a semi-circle. The right side of your back and your right shoulder will follow through with the rotation of your hips.

Finish with your hips squared to the front. Keep your left hand up and protect your face throughout.

Working on Your Punches

Practice definitely makes perfect when it comes to perfecting boxing moves. For this reason, the more time you put into practicing the correct way to throw a jab, cross, hook, and uppercut, the better. Not only will you learn the moves faster, you'll burn more calories, get into better shape faster, and develop a foundational blueprint for each basic punch.

Fortunately, you can practice your moves almost anytime and almost anywhere. There's no need to warm up or stretch because you can practice your punches at a safe, slow speed. What's more, you can perform all the basic moves in your street clothes, and you don't need any special equipment.

Whenever you have a free moment, throw an easy jab, punch, hook, or uppercut. After you've mastered the basic punches, use the DVD that comes with this book to customize your basic punches. Follow the instructor's cues—he is your personal trainer (on the DVD, that's yours truly). I will tell you to relax between punches and to hold your hands up. There will be gentle reminders to keep your elbows in and to focus on your imaginary opponent. Then begin practicing jab-cross-hook-uppercut combinations as presented on the DVD. Pause the DVD when necessary to correct your form.

Knockout Punch

If you're new to boxing, don't practice basic punches for more than 20 minutes at a time unless you're simply walking through the motions. These exercises use muscles that you probably haven't used before and it's easy to get overexcited and do too much too soon.

Not only do you train muscles when you launch your punches, but each time you complete your punch, you work muscles on the opposite side of your body. For example, every time you throw a jab or a cross you flex your chest and triceps. Just before your elbow reaches full extension, you stop the punch by contracting your back and biceps muscles.

Practicing the fundamentals will keep you in great shape. No matter how great you look, or how advanced you become, never neglect practicing the basic punches—they're what got you there.

The Least You Need to Know

◆ If you're new to boxing, keep your training sessions short. Under 20 minutes is best unless you're just practicing the moves. Form is more important than speed.

◆ Begin every punch in the basic fighting position—elbows in, chin down, hands up. Always relax and maintain your balance, and let your punches flow naturally.

◆ Boxing moves can, and should, be practiced often. Train whenever you get the chance.

◆ You don't have to punch fast and hard to master the moves. It's better to move with control as a beginner.

◆ Form is more important than speed and power. Practice in slow motion in front of a mirror.

In This Chapter

- ◆ Defense, defense!
- ◆ Staying on the move
- ◆ Bobbing and Weaving
- ◆ Ducking and Slipping

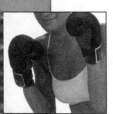
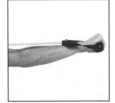
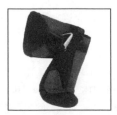
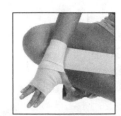
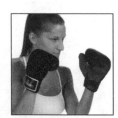
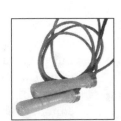

Chapter 13

Upper Body Moves

Defensive moves such as the Slip, the Duck, and the Bob and Weave protect boxers from the punches thrown by their opponents by leaving their hands free to counter their attacks.

They're great defensive moves for fitness boxers, too. Even better, they make for a fantastic abs and back workout, as they train these muscles at virtually every angle.

Moving All Around

When boxers aren't throwing punches, they're avoiding them. This requires almost constant movement that leaves the arms free to counterpunch. This constant movement not only burns calories, but it also moves your upper body at all angles and firms and tones your abs and back.

You'll have a tendency to over-exaggerate your movements in the beginning, but that's okay. The more inefficient your movements, the more calories you burn. With practice, your moves will be more efficient. You'll burn fewer calories unless you turn up the intensity, but your endurance will also be better.

Bending your knees and tilting at your waist are the movements responsible for changing your head position. Although boxers talk about head movement, if you do these moves correctly, your neck will barely move.

A well-balanced foundation is the key to your upper body movement. To change your vertical position, you'll bend your knees up and down. When you combine knee bends with tilting at the waist, you'll work many of the major muscle groups in your body.

Keep your hands up in a fighting position throughout these moves. Be careful not to drop your hands when you move your head.

Corner Man

To perform defensive moves correctly, try to imagine an opponent throwing a punch at you. This will intensify your effort and increase your calorie burn.

Everybody moves differently. You might not be able to Slip, and Bob and Weave like a prizefighter, but you can make the same moves on a much more subtle level and still reap substantial benefits from them.

Intersperse punches into your defensive drills. Slip and then throw a jab. Duck Under and then follow up with a right cross. Bob and Weave and then hook. The combinations are endless.

Everyone has a tendency to drop their hands when they practice defensive moves. Make a concerted effort to keep your hands up.

Slipping

It's often been said that the best defense is a good offense. In fitness boxing, the best way to block a punch, which is a defensive move, is not to be in its way in the first place. Slipping is one way to get out of the way of punches headed your way.

You slip a punch by bending at the waist and knees. In this way, the punch "slips" right past you. This move also leaves both of your hands free for counterpunching.

Tilt your upper body to the left or to the right to evade an imaginary punch to your face. Wait until you imagine the direction of the attack before you begin your movement.

Always use one hand to protect your face and the other to protect your midsection. Your partner may throw slow punches toward your face while you tilt your body out of the way.

Slipping a punch is a great way to tone up your midsection. The muscles of your abdominals contract when you tilt your body sideways.

Move slowly at first. After a few months, gradually pick up the pace. Keep your movements smooth without jerking your body from one side to the other.

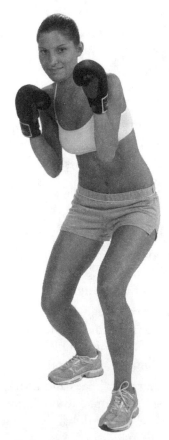

Keep a stable base with your hands up in a fighting position. Tilt your body to the right, maintaining a stable base. Keep your eyes on your imaginary opponent.

Be sure to move your entire upper body and not just your head and neck.

Duck Under

The Duck Under is a great bun and thigh toner, as your lower body should do most of the work.

Stand in a fighting position with your hands up and your upper body relaxed. Imagine someone throwing a hook punch at your head. Duck under the punch by bending at the knees while keeping your eyes focused on the solar plexus of your imaginary opponent.

Keep your hands up in a fighting position to reinforce your block, and don't bend your back. Resist the temptation to bend too much at the waist.

Knockout Punch

Be careful not to bend forward when you're doing defensive moves. Keeping your back straight when you execute them will help prevent lower back pain.

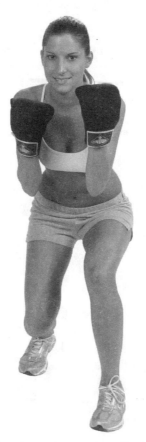

When you bend your knees, resist the temptation to drop your arms. Keep your back straight and your eyes up so you don't lose sight of your imaginary opponent.

Bob and Weave

The Bob and Weave tones your thighs, buns, and hamstrings. Move rhythmically from side to side. This is a great exercise to do to the beat of your favorite music.

Begin in a fighting position. Imagine your opponent punching at your head. Move to your left to avoid the punch. Then quickly bend your knees. Keep your hands up in a fighting position. When you come up again, shift to the right. Repeat.

Combine your Slip, Duck Under, and Bob and Weave moves into an awesome workout. Set your timer for 1-minute intervals and perform each movement for a minute. You can practice this 3-minute workout on your lunch break or use it as part of your overall fitness boxing program.

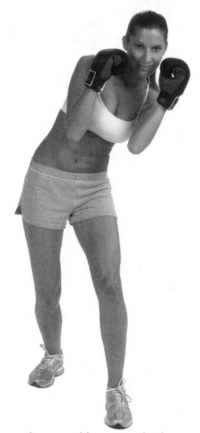

Bend your knees and keep your back straight just as you did during the Duck Under.

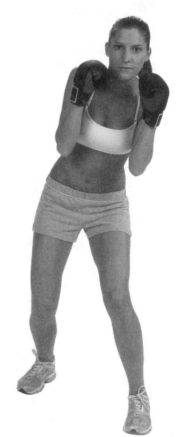

Keep your eyes up and tilt your entire upper body to the right to evade an imaginary punch.

Block

This drill is best done with a partner who's wearing target pads. Although you and your partner won't actually make contact, as there's no contact punching in fitness boxing, the target pads add to the ambiance and effectiveness of this exercise.

Using your arm to get in the way of an attack is instinctive, and following this instinct is exactly what you want to do. With your hands up and "tight," use the fist or outside portion of the wrist to block a headshot. Use the elbow or forearm to block a body punch. This technique works best against long, hooking shots.

The Least You Need to Know

◆ Defensive moves such as Slipping and Bobbing and Weaving are natural ab and back exercises. The bending and twisting required firms and tones your torso and strengthens your abs and back.

◆ Keep your hands up no matter where your body is.

◆ If the move doesn't feel right, don't do it. Slipping and Bobbing and Weaving can strain your back. Stay with the moves that feel comfortable.

◆ Don't bend forward when you do defensive moves. Keep your back straight to help prevent lower back pain.

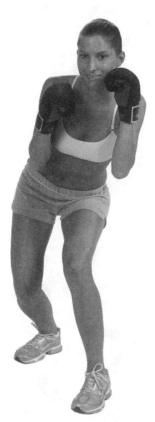

Keep your arm close to your body and imagine your opponent hitting your arm.

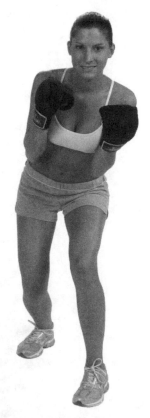

Be sure your hands stay up next to your face and your arm touches your ribs. Block the punch by moving it aside. Redirect the punch smoothly instead of striking at it.

In This Chapter

- ◆ Using bands for speed and strength
- ◆ Tips for working with bands
- ◆ Punching with resistance
- ◆ Training fast, training slow
- ◆ Working out safely

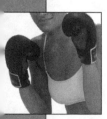
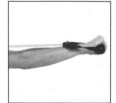
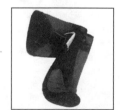
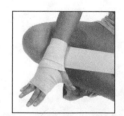
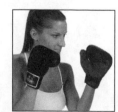
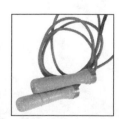

Boxing With Bands

Boxers use exercise bands to develop speed and strength so they can deliver punches when they're closer to their opponents than they'd like to be. The ideal distance—an arm's length away—allows maximum power in each punch, and is something that opponents try to make sure doesn't happen. Instead, they move around to ensure the shortest angle, which lessens or eliminates any mechanical advantage.

Fitness boxing borrowed their exercises, not necessarily to gain an advantage over their opponents, but because the moves are very effective for building strength, speed, and power. They also firm and tone hard-to-reach balancing muscles.

Band training is a safe and user-friendly way to practice punches at full speed with resistance. It's also good for toning, shaping, and firming your entire body.

Advantages to Fitness Band Training

Exercise bands can be used to punch at variable speeds and angles. You can train one muscle group at a time or several in unison.

Knowing that you have to slow down at the end of a lift or a punch limits your strength and the ability to fully tone your muscles because you decelerate—in other words, you don't keep going through the move. You can liken it to forgetting to wear your hand wraps and being afraid you'll hurt your hands when you hit the heavy bag. You wouldn't hit the bag with everything you had; you'd "pull your punches." In other words, you'd decelerate just before you made contact with the bag to avoid injury.

Using exercise bands helps you move as fast as you can through your entire range of motion on each punch. There's no need to slow down at the end because you're not hitting anything. You can throw repetitive punches without fear of injury.

Why punch with fitness bands instead of just shadowboxing? Punching against resistance uses more muscle fibers; for example, more muscles firm up faster. Shadowboxing can make you fast by throwing hundreds of punches in the air, but it doesn't necessarily develop the strength needed for punching properly. Instead of generating true power from your body, you "arm punch." This can put unnecessary strain on your rotator cuffs, and lead to injury.

Exercise band training also lets you train for strength, endurance, flexibility, balance, and power all at once without requiring extra time in the gym. As the band stretches out, the exercise gets harder. Unlike free weights where after you start the weight moving, momentum takes over; the further you stretch the exercise band, the more resistance you will feel.

Bands require you to punch with resistance, and the added resistance will slow down your punches at first. As you get stronger, you'll adapt to the resistance and punch faster. The more powerful you become, the less chance you have of incurring an injury. When you train without the bands, your moves will seem easier because they are, and you will be that much faster.

The ability to produce maximal force (for example, muscular strength) and the ability to achieve great velocity in the same motion are different motor abilities. That's why exercise bands help you train for both within the same movement. They increase your quickness and reaction time, and improve your speed and power—the interaction between strength and speed.

Preparing for Band Training

Band training can be done individually or with a partner. If you're working out by yourself and you're doing moves that call for the band to be anchored by anything other than your feet or your other hand, you'll have to attach it to something. Ballet bars or hooks are options;

there are also special strap attachments you can buy that will let you anchor the band in a door jam. Always check the security of the attachment before performing any band exercise.

> **Knockout Punch**
>
> Don't anchor a band by shutting it in-between a door and a door jam. This can damage the band and cause it to wear out quickly. Tying a band to a doorknob isn't a good idea, either. It too can lead to early breaking, not to mention possible injury to you or damage to the interior of your house should you pull the door open.

Partner training with bands is great because both you and your partner get a great workout. When you practice band drills with a partner, your partner holds the end of the band and vice versa. Just holding the bands is a workout in itself because you have to provide resistance while maintaining your balance. Be sure that if a friend holds the band for you he or she doesn't think there's anything funny about letting go in the middle of your routine. This could lead to serious injury for both of you.

Always visually inspect your bands for wear before you start a band training routine. There's nothing worse than the sound of a band snapping in half in the middle of an exercise. Look for small cracks, tears, or abrasions. They'll typically show up in areas where you've anchored the band to something. If you find visible wear, get a new band. Don't risk using your old one—it could snap at any time.

More exercise band training tips:

- ◆ Grab your fitness band firmly. When you make a fist, be sure to roll your fingers tightly around the band or handle to protect your hands. Press your thumbs tightly against your index and middle fingers on the outside of your fist. Keep your elbows slightly bent (soft) on all punches and strikes.

◆ When you punch, begin slowly. Move through a full range of motion on each technique. At first pay attention to form without concern about overall performance.

◆ Move through the exact range of motion required. If you don't train your muscles along the correct line of pull, you'll lose many of the benefits of the exercise.

◆ If twisting movements don't feel right, choose a different exercise. If you feel any discomfort on an exercise, try doing it from a slightly different angle.

Knockout Punch

Band training can feel like a fairly lightweight workout, but it's definitely not. Be careful to begin slowly and progress gradually to prevent sore muscles. Soon you'll be able to punch with the same speed as you did without the bands.

As you get accustomed to using the bands, you can decide how fast you want to punch with them. Your rate of speed depends on how you train. If you train for speed, you will get faster. If you train slow, you will stay slow. High-speed training with moderate resistance provides increased strength, power, and muscle definition.

If you train for speed, be sure to maintain form. You can move your exercise band very quickly, but always keep your movements under control.

A band workout that tones all the muscles in your body can be accomplished in as little as 30 minutes. Begin with a 6-minute warm-up combining 2 minutes of the Boxer's Shuffle with Lateral Resistance and 2 minutes of the Boxer's Shuffle with Posterior Resistance. Be sure to switch sides on your Boxer's Shuffle with Lateral Resistance after the first 2 minutes. Anchor the band at waist level.

Here's a sample 30-minute band workout. Since the short workout below does not involve all of the band exercises in this chapter, feel free to mix and match the remaining band exercises into a program that fits your needs, goals, and schedule:

Boxer's Shuffle with Lateral Resistance (right side)—2 minutes

Boxer's Shuffle with Lateral Resistance (left side)—2 minutes

Boxer's Shuffle with Posterior Resistance—2 minutes

Chop Wood Like a Boxer—5 minutes. Concentrate on correct form by keeping your abs tight and your back straight. Anchor the band at head level.

Without rest, begin Rapid Single Arm Push with Resistance. Keep your torso tight and twist your body and your arm into each punch. Switch hands after each minute. Perform three sets with each arm for a total of six sets in 6 minutes. Anchor the band at waist level.

You're more than halfway through your workout, but don't take a break. Grab your bands with both hands and perform Cross Pull with Resistance. Switch sides after each minute. Perform three sets on each side for a total of six sets in 6 minutes. The band remains anchored at waist level.

Finish up with Ankle Strap, Opposite Leg Balance with Resistance. Secure the band around your ankle and focus on the balance and strength of your lower body. Perform 2 minutes of Ankle Strap, Opposite Leg Balance with each leg.

Cool down for the final 3 minutes with easy shadowboxing. Without resistance, your arms and legs should feel strong and fast. Be careful to pace yourself. Move slowly and remember that this is your relaxing cool down.

If twisting movements don't feel right, choose a different exercise. Find a slightly different angle to do an exercise if you feel discomfort.

Boxer's Shuffle with Lateral Resistance

This exercise trains all the muscles in your lower body. It especially tones and firms the difficult-to-target inner and outer thigh muscles.

Secure the band on your hand in the fighting position. Perform the Boxer's Shuffle sideways pulling away from the resistance.

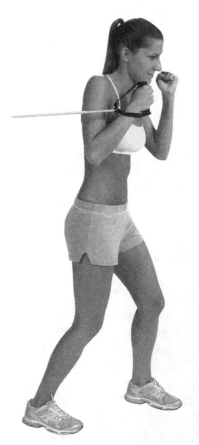

Maintain correct posture although you will feel the band pulling from the side.

Boxer's Shuffle with Posterior Resistance

This exercise firms and tones the thighs and buns.

Secure the band on the back of your hip. Perform the Boxer's Shuffle. The added resistance challenges your thighs and buns. Adding resistance to the Boxer's Shuffle accelerates your progress so that you'll see noticeable results in a shorter period than if you performed the Boxer's Shuffle without resistance.

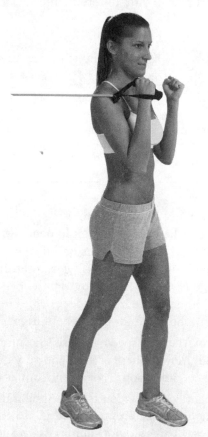

Keep your back straight and abs tight as you feel the pull from the back.

Chop Wood Like a Boxer (High to Low)

This is a full-body exercise that tones and strengthens the calves, thighs, buns, waist, shoulders, and arms.

Grab one end of the band with both hands. Begin with the band held over your shoulder. Your partner holds the band high so that you feel the resistance on the way down.

Corner Man

On all "chopping exercises," be careful to protect your back by keeping your abdominals tight and your back straight.

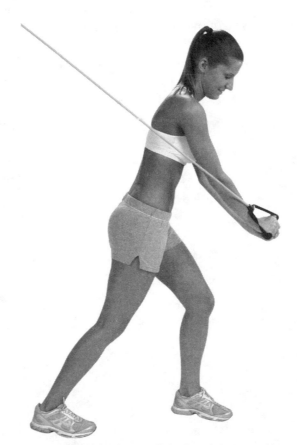

Use your whole body to pull the band down to the low position.

Rapid Single Arm Push with Resistance

This exercise firms and tones the buns, waist, chest, and arms.

Begin in a fighting stance with the handle of one end of the exercise band in your left hand. Punch with your left hand out to the front. The palm of your left hand should face the floor. Retract your left hand to the fighting position as quickly as you can and repeat punches in a piston-like motion, striking with the first two knuckles.

Pushing your punch, which means that you use your arm instead of your body to create power, is something that many beginning fitness boxers fall into a bad habit of doing. Learn to relax so your arms feel like strings with fists attached. Keep your knees bent and your back straight in a solid fighting stance.

Notice that the power begins in your hips and moves through the chest, shoulder, elbow, wrist, and finally blasts through the fist. Your legs are a stable base, providing a foundation and generating force outward through your hand.

Take this powerful application into your fitness boxing workout. Not only will you develop strong, powerful punches, but you will expend more energy and trim and firm your entire body. Switch arms and repeat.

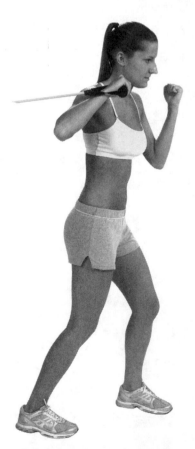

Begin in a fighting position with your arm ready to punch. Be sure there is no slack in the exercise band.

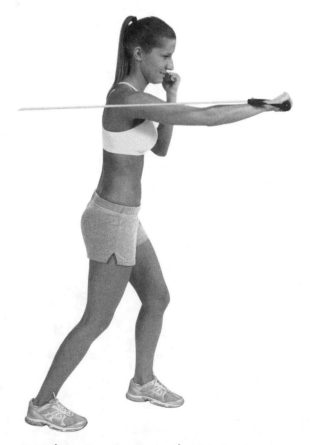

Extend your arm as you punch against resistance. Keep your back straight and your abs tight.

Reverse Follow Through with Resistance

Your partner holds the band behind you at head level. Hold the handle in your hand and extend your right arm out in front as if you had completed a punch. Cock your right arm back in a throwing motion. Switch arms and repeat.

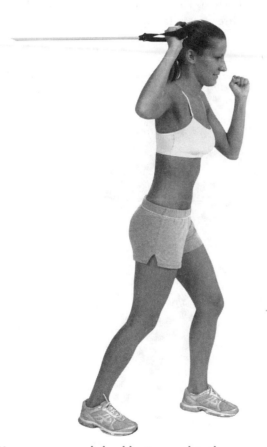

Use your arm and shoulder to complete the move. Keep your abs tight.

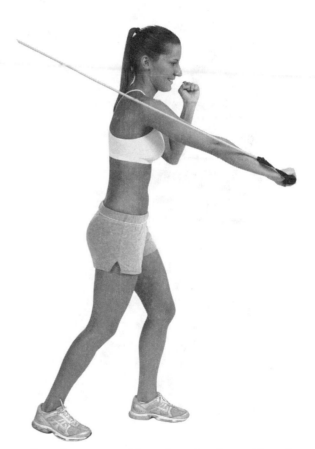

Extend your arm without changing the position of your lower body.

Cross Pull with Resistance

Hold the handles in both hands in front of your body. Twist your body to the right. Switch sides and repeat.

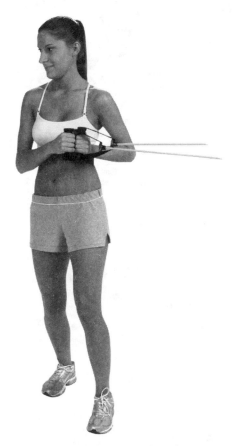

Contract the muscles on the sides of your waist to twist your body. Keep your back straight and arms relaxed.

Cross Pull, Leg Balance with Resistance

Lift your right foot off the floor. Hold the handles in both hands in front of your body. Twist your body to the right. Switch sides and repeat. Then lift your left foot off the floor and repeat.

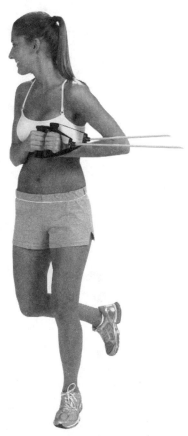

Perform the same movement as the cross pull. You'll use your stabilizer muscles to keep your balance.

Front Punch Push with Resistance

Hold a handle in one hand while your partner holds the other end behind you. Retract each arm back and forth.

Use your whole body to complete the punch beginning with the pivot of your foot.

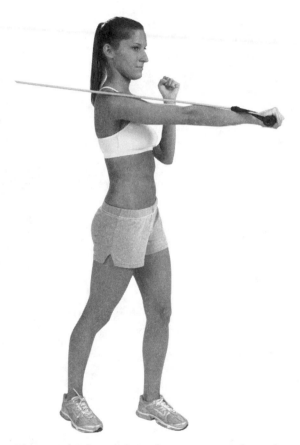

Keep your back straight and contract your abs at the completion of your punch.

Stable Body, Punching with Resistance

Stand with your body motionless and use your right arm to punch. Switch hands and repeat. Your core must stabilize your movement.

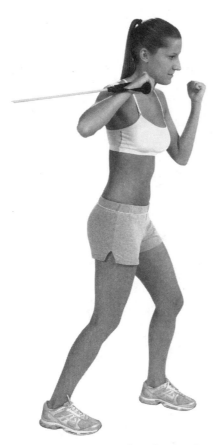

Use your arm to complete the punch.

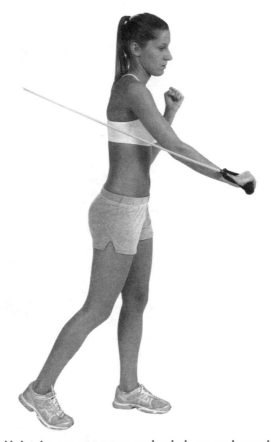

Maintain correct posture and exhale on each punch.

Ankle Strap, Opposite Leg Balance with Resistance

This exercise firms and tones stabilizer muscles in your waist and hips.

Place one of the handles around your right ankle. Keep your hands up in a fighting position and raise your right foot a few inches off the floor. Hold this pose. The resistance that is applied to your right side forces stabilizer muscles to fire throughout your waist and hips. Switch legs and repeat.

The Least You Need to Know

◆ Band training allows you to practice your punches at full speed with resistance. It's a safe, user-friendly way to tone, shape, and firm up your entire body.

◆ Always check your bands for excessive wear before starting an exercise band workout.

◆ Move through the exact range of motion required. If you don't train your muscles along the correct line of pull, you'll lose many of the strength and toning benefits.

◆ Always keep your movements under control when training with bands. If you train for speed, be sure to maintain correct form.

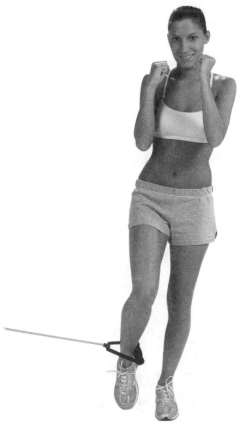

Your body must fight the resistance band by maintaining correct posture.

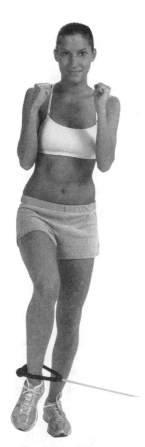

Try to be absolutely still throughout the duration of this exercise.

In This Chapter

- ◆ Building a fitness boxing foundation
- ◆ Increasing quickness and endurance
- ◆ The best shoes for footwork drills
- ◆ Fabulous footwork drills

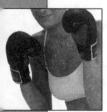
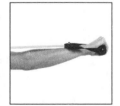
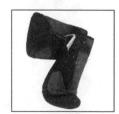
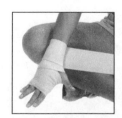
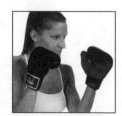
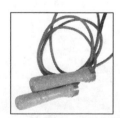

Fancy Footwork

Boxers in the ring almost never stand still. Nor do good fitness boxers. Good footwork is essential for making the most of boxing moves, whether in the ring or when using them in fitness boxing routines.

In this chapter, you learn principles of boxing footwork that will keep you light on your feet throughout your fitness boxing workouts.

Footing Your Foundation

Footwork is the foundation for fitness boxing, just like it is for boxing in the ring. All punches and blocks rely on a firm base of support in the lower body that's created by keeping your body centered and balanced at all times. A firm base also helps maintain your fighting stance no matter what direction you're moving in—forward, backward, side-to-side, at an angle, around your opponent, you name it.

Agility—staying light on the balls of your feet—is also necessary. Footwork drills accomplish both. What's more, footwork drills are a great workout for your lower body—thighs, hamstrings, and buns. Because you're keeping the larger muscles of your lower body moving constantly when you do these drills, you also fire up your metabolic furnace in a big way.

Footwork drills increase your quickness and endurance. If you haven't done them before, be prepared for a steep learning curve—they aren't easy! Keep doing them, and you'll be amazed at how quickly your feet take on a life of their own.

Footwork drills are also good to do if your upper body is sore, as you don't have to pair these drills with an upper body workout.

Sweet Science

Footwork training involves small steps back and to the side, circling an imaginary opponent, and quick in and out movements. You keep moving all the time—when you're hitting focus mitts, a heavy bag, and when sparring or shadowboxing. With practice, your footwork becomes fluid, relaxed, efficient, and balanced.

Always be sure to warm up thoroughly before doing footwork drills. These drills use both large and small muscles in your lower body. Concentrate on staying on the balls of your feet.

Starting on the Right Foot

The boxer's stance is the starting point for all boxing moves, and is also the position you want to be in for footwork drills. If your boxer's stance isn't correct, it's difficult to perform moves safely and effectively, so let's review it again:

◆ Position your feet comfortably apart, with your weight more toward the balls of your feet. Your weight should be evenly balanced between your feet. You should feel balanced and able to move easily. Be sure to keep your knees bent, but not too deeply.

◆ Turn slightly sideways to your imaginary opponent. Your front foot, hip, and shoulders should all be aligned. Keep the top of your left fist aligned with the top of your shoulders. Extend your elbow slightly but be sure to keep it close to your body for protection.

◆ Keep your right fist close to your chin. Your right elbow should remain close to your ribs.

◆ Relax your neck and shoulders. Make sure you're not hunching your shoulders up to your ears.

When you're in this position, test your balance by rocking back and forth lightly from foot to foot. Your heels should lightly touch the floor; most of your weight should be on the balls of your feet.

Keep your body in the proper fighting position when practicing all your footwork drills. Keep your hands up and your knees and elbows slightly bent (soft) during your entire workout.

Knockout Punch

Don't crouch too low when you bend your knees in a boxer's stance. Doing so can be awkward and will tire you out quickly.

If possible, check your alignment and posture in a mirror: eyes straight ahead, back straight, shoulder blades pulled back, top of your shoulders parallel, stomach in, and knees and shoulders soft. Do this as often as you need to. Your body will eventually remember what this position feels like so you'll be able to assume it automatically. Until then, it's a good idea to keep an eye—literally—on how you're doing things.

Using a mirror to check your form when you do footwork drills is a good idea. Or you can do them with a partner.

Footwear for Footwork

You can wear the same shoes you use for your other workouts when you do footwork drills. Just make sure they provide enough stabilization and support for your individual movement style. Or try a boxing shoe. Because boxing footwork requires shuffling, pivoting, and quick feet, a light shoe with a flat bottom is optimal, and a boxing shoe is built this way.

If you need new shoes, visit a shoe store such as Foot Locker that specializes in fitting you with the proper shoe for your foot. Have the sales person watch you walk, and bring along a pair of shoes so he or she can see the wear pattern on them. Both will indicate the kind of shoe you need—maybe one with motion control or perhaps one with a higher arch for better support.

Basic Shuffle Moves

The general rule of movement in the ring is to first move the foot that is closest to the direction in which you want to go. The general rule of movement when fitness boxing is the same thing—your first move will be the foot closest to the direction you want to go.

For example, if you want to move forward, step with your front foot and follow with your back foot. If you want to move to the left, step first with your left foot and follow it with your right foot.

One fun footwork pattern that you might enjoy practicing is a combination of the Forward Shuffle, Backward Shuffle, Lateral Shuffle, and Ali Shuffle. All you need is about five square feet of floor space to perform this routine. Start in a fighting position on the balls of your feet. Shuffle forward as quickly as you can. Stay light on your feet and hold this position for a count of three (3 seconds). Then shuffle backward so that you wind up in your original position. Your hands remain in a fighting position and you stay level throughout your movement. Hold for 3 seconds.

Now perform a Lateral Shuffle to the left and hold for 3 seconds. Follow this with a Lateral Shuffle to the right. Hold for 3 seconds.

The final move is the Ali Shuffle. After you complete it, hold for 3 seconds and begin the entire sequence again.

Your goal is to complete the entire cycle 10 times. When you can, add two cycles per week until you can perform 18 consecutive cycles.

Boxer's Forward Shuffle

The Boxer's Forward Shuffle uses the large muscle groups in your legs and is a great fat burner for that reason. Not only do your calves, quads, hamstrings, and buns work to move you forward, the muscles on the inside and outside of your legs also work to balance your movements.

Begin in a fighting stance. Slide your front foot forward about 6 inches. Let your back foot slide up to replace your front foot. Do this as quickly as you can. Keep your shoulders and hips level throughout. Your knees should be bent at all times.

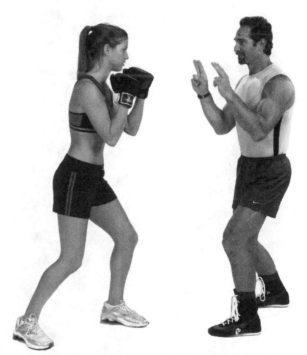

Push off the ball of your right foot as you step forward with your left foot. Pull the right foot up to replace the position of your left foot.

Corner Man

Exhale through pursed lips on each movement of your footwork pattern. A strong exhalation tightens your abs and keeps you in the boxing mindset.

⊙ Boxer's Backward Shuffle

Perform a Boxer's Backward Shuffle to retreat by sliding your back foot backward 6 inches and allow your front foot to replace it. Be sure that your hands remain in a fighting position throughout the shuffle.

Keep both knees bent so you stay level. Keep you upper body relaxed and stay on the balls of your feet. Move quickly and effortlessly exhaling through pursed lips.

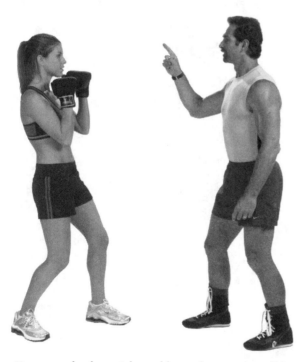

Keep your back straight and knees bent as you slide your right foot back and your left foot follows.

Boxer's Lateral Shuffle

The Boxer's Lateral Shuffle strengthens and tones your inner and outer thigh muscles. Exhale into each move just as you did for the forward and backward shuffles.

If you move to your left, push off your right foot and slide your left foot into position. To move to your right, push off your left foot and slide your right foot into position.

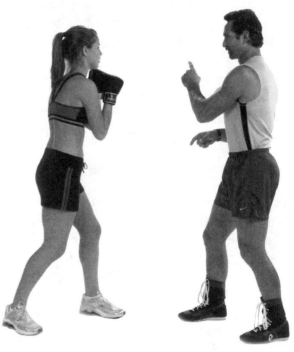

Keep your upper body relaxed with your hands up. Stay level by keeping your knees bent throughout the movement.

Boxer's Angular Shuffle

The Boxer's Angular Shuffle, which uses a lot of muscles that don't get much action during a typical workout, firms and tones your outer and inner thigh muscles.

Use the same footwork as the Boxer's Shuffle to move at different oblique angles instead of simply forward or backward. You can move at a 45-degree angle to the front or to the back. Exhale on each move.

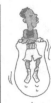

Sweet Science

Humans aren't robots. We're not made to only move in a linear direction. Moving at different angles uses a variety of muscles you didn't know you had until you feel them the next day.

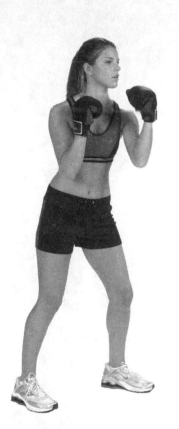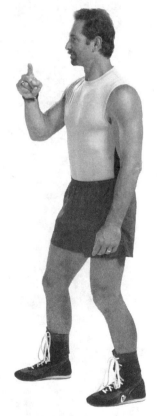

Stay light on the balls of your feet and remain level throughout the Angular Shuffle.

Ali Shuffle

The Ali Shuffle firms and tones all the muscles in your legs and if performed in repetition, is an excellent fat burner.

The Ali Shuffle is named for the famous quick-stepping footwork pattern of world heavyweight champion Muhammad Ali. Ali's fancy footwork outwitted some of the most formidable challengers of his era. The Ali Shuffle requires a lot of energy so it's a great fat burner. Stay on the balls of your feet and keep your feet pointing in the same direction throughout as if you were on a cross-country ski machine.

Begin in a left foot forward fighting stance. Twist your hips quickly and switch your feet into a right foot forward fighting stance. Your feet should barely leave the floor and then they should move right back to their original position. Your shoulders and hips should remain level throughout. Your eyes are on your imaginary opponent.

At first, the Ali Shuffle may feel very difficult. If so, break the movement in half. Perform half the shuffle, take a few seconds rest, and then complete the other half. Take a few seconds between to rest if you're performing reps.

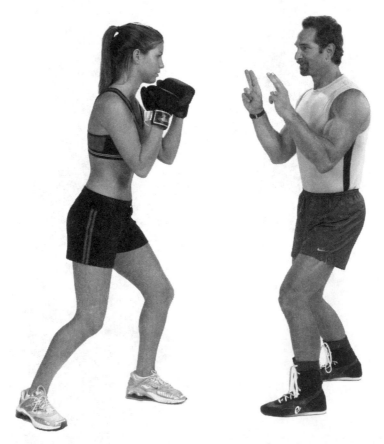

Although both feet leave the floor for a split second, keep your feet as close to the floor as possible.

If your calves can't handle the strain of remaining on the balls of your feet throughout the workout, drop your heels occasionally when performing certain punches and blocks. This will give your calves the chance to rest a few seconds between exercise sets.

The Least You Need to Know

- Footwork is your foundation for fitness boxing. All punches and blocks rely on a firm lower body base of support.

- Fancy footwork burns fat. Constant lower body movement burns a tremendous amount of calories, which translates into a great fat-burning workout.

- Your lower body uses more muscle than your upper body. Thighs, hamstrings, and buns make up significantly more muscle than your upper body. This means there's more potential for increasing your metabolic furnace.

- Footwork drills increase your quickness and endurance. You'll be amazed at how quickly your feet take on a life of their own. Because you may not have practiced footwork drills before, the learning curve is steep.

- If your upper body is sore, do footwork drills. Footwork drills may be practiced without upper body work. Concentrate on staying on the balls of your feet.

- Warm up thoroughly before footwork drills. Footwork drills use both large and small muscles in your lower body. They must be warmed up before you proceed.

In This Chapter

- ◆ Boxing combos
- ◆ Putting your punches together
- ◆ Practicing form, then speed
- ◆ The best combo workouts

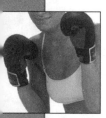 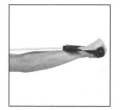 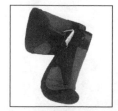 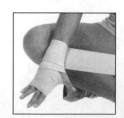 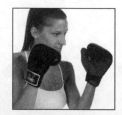 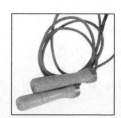

Chapter 16

Stinging Like a Bee

Putting your punches together into combinations is the complete fitness boxing workout. It's the real deal—you're combining everything you know about punches, footwork, and timing into a full-fledged boxing workout. Not only are you working out like a boxer, you look like a boxer when you do them.

Combos also add a new level of difficulty and intensity to your workouts and help improve your coordination and agility. Plus, there's nothing like the feeling of accomplishment when you can throw rapid-fire combinations without even thinking about them.

First Comes Form

Practice makes perfect no matter what you do, but it's ultra important when it comes to punching combos. It takes thousands of repetitions to perfect jabs, hooks, and uppercuts, and thousands more to get them to where they look and feel natural.

Repetition is the best way to perfect your punching power. But it's important to practice correctly, which means keeping your form as perfect as possible. Move slowly and concentrate on your form until combinations feel natural to you. It's better to practice 1 repetition with correct form than to practice 1,000 repetitions incorrectly.

Then Comes Speed

Power is a combination of strength and speed. For a punch to be powerful, it must have both force (strength) and speed. Force is the muscle behind your punch. Speed is how fast you can move your muscles. It's a combination of reaction time and movement time. Reaction time is measured from the moment you think about executing a technique until you actually move your muscles.

Try an experiment. Throw a jab-cross-hook combination very slowly. Concentrate on your form. Monitor your breathing and your effort. Now, throw a jab-cross-hook combination with speed and power. Notice the difference in your breathing. These fast, powerful punching combinations take more effort. Consequently, they burn tons of calories.

The more muscle you possess, the more powerful you become. But you still have to learn how to move your muscles correctly to develop speed.

At first, throw your combinations slowly so you can learn the movements. When you can throw your combinations efficiently, add a little speed. As you improve your reaction time and movement time, the speed and power of your punching combinations will also improve. You'll be able to throw more punches in a shorter period of time and get a more strenuous workout.

Sweet Science

Form is paramount when practicing combinations. When you can throw your combinations efficiently, add a little speed. The faster and more powerful you can make your movements, the more you'll stoke your metabolic furnace.

Here are some combo workout tips:

◆ Let your combinations flow one to the next. Stay smooth and relaxed. Avoid doing fast, jerky motions.

◆ Throw complete moves rather than rushing through each combination. Someone watching you should not have to guess which punches and defensive moves you're doing.

◆ Always keep one hand next to your face. A good way to do this is to make light contact with your hand on the side of your cheek.

◆ If you're practicing without a partner, imagine an opponent in front of you. An imaginary opponent increases your energy level, burns more calories, and improves your workout.

◆ Keep your feet moving at all times. Never stop. Stay light on your feet. Always be a moving target. Doing so will burn more calories and improve the shape of your calf muscles.

◆ Maintain tight abs and a relaxed upper body throughout. With relaxation comes speed and with correct posture you will lower your risk of an injury.

Double Jab

Start with your left leg forward in a fighting stance. Step forward with your left foot and execute two consecutive jabs with your left hand.

Exhale on each jab and be sure to bring your left hand back into a fighting position immediately upon execution. Get your shoulder into each punch and don't try to punch too hard. Form is more important than speed and power.

Your triceps muscles extend your arm and your biceps bring it back to a fighting position. Doing Double Jabs will increase the tone and definition in both your triceps and biceps muscles.

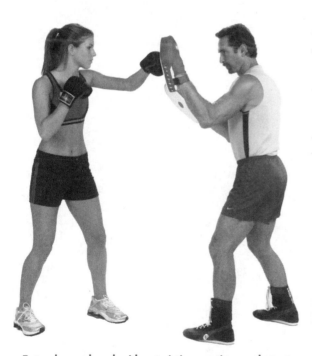

Extend your hand with a twisting motion so that at contact with a pad, bag, imaginary or real opponent, your palm is pointing down. Retract your hand and extend it again like a piston. Use your shoulder to power each punch.

Jab, Cross

The Left Jab, Right Cross combination works most of the muscles in your body. Stepping into the jab and pivoting into the cross firms and tones your lower body muscles. When you extend your shoulder into your jab and twist your torso into your cross, you fire all the muscles in your abs, back, shoulders, and arms.

Start with your left leg forward in a fighting stance. Step forward with your left foot and simultaneously throw a Left Jab. Retract your jab, immediately move back into a fighting position, and then throw a Right Cross.

Pause between the jab and the cross until your form is perfect. Take your time and exhale on each punch. When you throw your cross, start your movement with a pivot of your right foot. Be sure to keep your left hand in a fighting position until you complete the Right Cross.

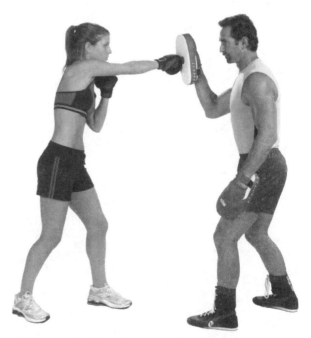

Keep your back straight and imagine you're shooting your jab out of the barrel of a gun. Pivot your right foot into the cross so that a power chain emanates from your foot and travels through your hips, abs, shoulders, and arms.

Jab, Cross, Hook

Twisting your torso back and forth as this drill requires is a vigorous, calorie-burning work-out. Your triceps, back, shoulders, chest, waist, and hips are all recruited during this exercise.

Start with your left leg forward in a fighting stance. Step forward with your left foot and simultaneously throw a Left Jab. Retract your jab and immediately throw a Right Cross. Then follow up with a Left Hook.

Move through each punch as a single move at first. Take your time and concentrate on your form—step into your jab with your left foot, pivot your right foot into your cross, pivot your left foot into your hook.

There is a whole-body twisting effect that occurs when you throw each of the punches. When you alternate hands for the jab, cross, hook, you create a powerful stretch-release action from one move to the next.

The power in each punch is magnified by the punch preceding it. The Right Cross gets its power from the reciprocal motion created from pulling back the Left Jab. And the Left Hook receives some added zing from the retraction of the Right Cross.

At first when you do this combination, it might feel like your body is working against itself. After you've practiced this combination for several months, you'll amaze yourself with your new-found efficiency and finesse. In the words of heavyweight boxer Muhammad Ali's corner man, you will "float like a butterfly and sting like a bee."

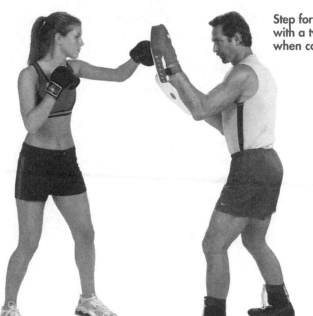

Step forward with your left foot and extend your left hand with a twisting motion so that your palm is pointing down when contact is reached with your imaginary opponent.

Retract your left hand back to a fighting position and pivot your right foot into a cross so that a power chain moves from your foot through your hips, abs, shoulders, and arms.

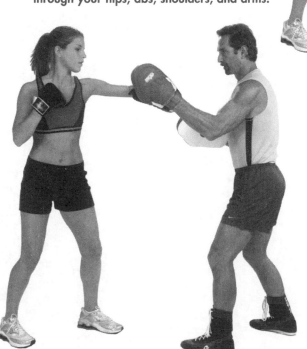

Retract your right arm and pivot your left foot inward. Simultaneously move your left forearm parallel to the floor and follow through with a Left Hook.

Jab, Cross, Hook, Uppercut

This four-step combination feels like a marathon. You actually may feel winded after a couple of reps. Pace yourself and move slowly at first. Then gradually pick up the pace. Soon you'll be able to perform all four punches without thinking. That's when you know you're looking good.

Break this combination into four separate punches—step and jab, twist and cross, pivot and hook, bend and uppercut. Pause between each technique and check your form in the mirror. Be sure not to rush. Instead be meticulous, executing each technique as if it were the only one you were concerned with.

Start with your left leg forward in a fighting stance. Step forward with your left foot and simultaneously throw a Left Jab. Retract your jab and immediately throw a Right Cross. Then immediately follow up with a Left Hook.

Finally, bend your knees and keep your elbows into your side as you throw a finishing Right Uppercut.

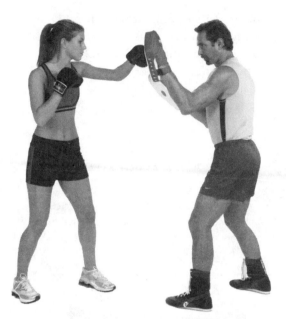

Keep your back straight. Imagine that you're shooting your jab out of the barrel of a gun.

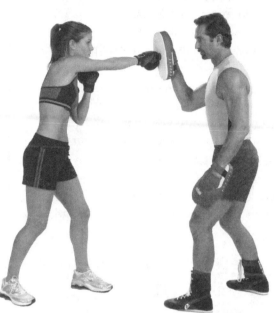

As soon as you retract your jab, begin pivoting on your right foot in preparation for your Right Cross.

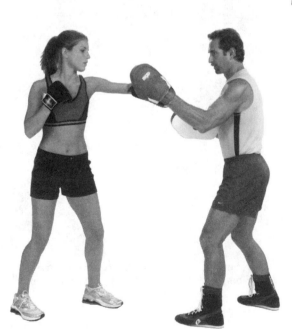

Pivot on your left foot and twist from your hip and waist to complete your Left Hook.

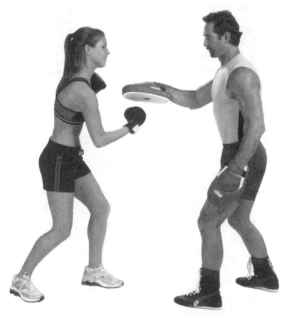

Bend from your knees and hips while you keep your right elbow bent at 90 degrees. Launch your Right Uppercut from your hip propelling your punch upward toward your imaginary target.

Jab, Hook

Start with your left leg forward in a fighting stance. Step forward with your left foot and execute a Left Jab. As soon as you retract your jab to your original fighting stance position, throw a Left Hook. Switch sides and repeat.

If you do this combination incorrectly, you'll be throwing arm punches. Instead, get your body weight into your Left Jab by stepping forward with your left foot and turning your left shoulder slightly inward.

As soon as you complete your jab, retract your hand back to a fighting position. Immediately pivot on the ball of your left foot and begin the power surge that travels from your foot, through your hip, waist, and chest, and out your arm into your fist. Return back into a fighting position.

The jab, hook firms and tones the muscles of your chest, arms, torso, and legs.

Knockout Punch

Be careful not to swing wide on your hook as doing so can strain the muscles in your shoulders. Instead keep your hook tight, close to your body, and compact.

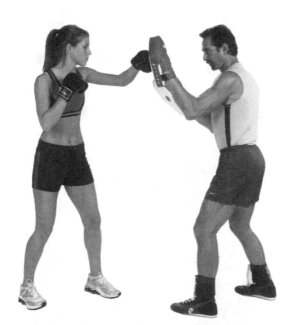

Step forward into your Left Jab keeping your back straight and elbows soft.

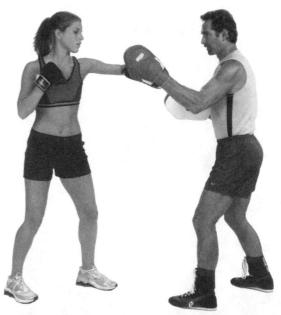

Pivot on the ball of your left foot keeping your elbow bent at 90 degrees and your forearm parallel to the floor.

Double Hook

The Double Hook trains muscles on the entire left side of your body.

Begin in a fighting stance and step forward with your left foot while simultaneously throwing a Left Hook. Keep your right hand up in a fighting position. Immediately throw another Left Hook.

Throwing two consecutive Left Hooks is quite a demanding exercise. The left side of your waist and hips are required to work double-duty without the usual stretch-recovery cycle that occurs when you throw a jab, cross.

For this reason, be careful not to overtrain your Double Hook during each fitness boxing workout. Instead, intersperse your Double Hooks with other combinations that include crosses and uppercuts.

Corner Man

Using your lower body, such as in the Duck Under, burns about twice as many calories as a simple punch. Include bobs, weaves, and the Duck Under into your repertoire to accelerate fat loss.

Cross, Hook

The cross, hook is a combination of two power punches. Both the cross and the hook use your entire body to create power.

Throw a Right Cross straight to the head of your imaginary opponent. Keep your left hand up in a fighting position. At the moment you complete your Right Cross, pivot on the balls of your feet in the other direction and complete a Left Hook.

Use that rubberband-like effect after you throw your cross to power your hook. First your body twists to the left when you throw the cross. Then it rebounds to the right when you execute your hook.

All your ab muscles contract when you perform this combination.

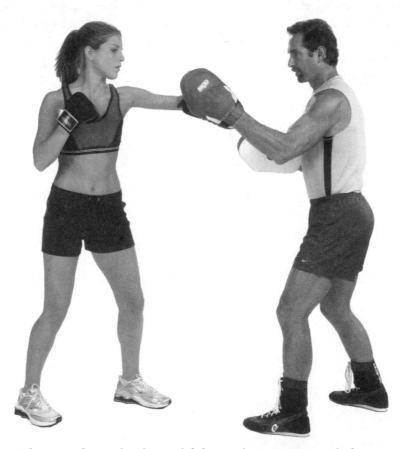

Take a step forward with your left foot and pivot on your right foot as you execute a Right Cross. As soon as you complete the cross, bring your hands back into a fighting position and without hesitation, pivot on your left foot and complete your hook.

💿 Jab, Bob and Weave, Hook

This exercise combines an attack with a defensive move, then another attack. It's a very vigorous combination that, when perfected, makes you really look like a boxer.

Throw a Left Jab and imagine your opponent is countering with a Right Cross. Bob and Weave under the imaginary cross, pivot on the balls of your feet, and complete a Left Hook.

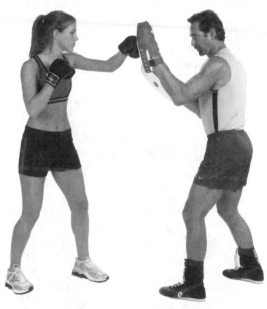

Step forward with your left foot and throw a Left Jab. Keep your back straight.

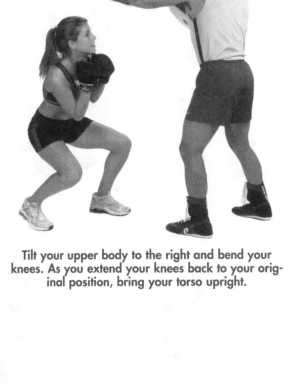

Tilt your upper body to the right and bend your knees. As you extend your knees back to your original position, bring your torso upright.

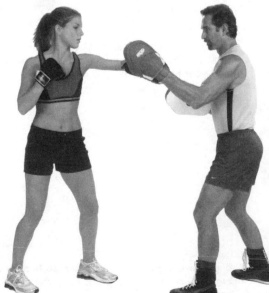

When you reach your original fighting stance position, pivot inward on the ball of your left foot and execute a Left Hook.

Jab, Bob and Weave, Cross

This is another full-body offensive and defensive combo. All your muscles work together in synchronous harmony to complete this move.

Throw a Left Jab and imagine your opponent is countering with a Right Cross. Bob and Weave under the imaginary cross and pivot on the balls of your feet and complete a Right Cross.

Try to stay light on your feet and examine your form in the mirror to maintain a smooth flow between one movement and the next.

Keep your elbows in, hands up, and chin down. Execute a Left Jab and return your hand back to a fighting position immediately.

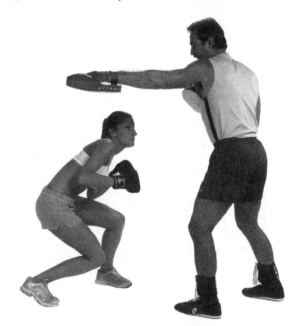

As soon as you complete your jab, duck straight down by bending your knees and hips. As you extend your knees, come up a few inches to your right.

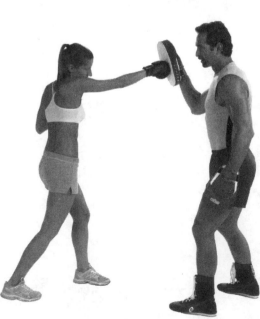

Begin pivoting on your right foot so that by the time you're in a fighting position, you may complete your Right Cross.

The Least You Need to Know

◆ Putting your punches together into combinations is the real deal—you're combining everything you know about punches, footwork, and timing into a full-fledged boxing workout.

◆ Start slowly. Perfect your moves, and then work on speed.

◆ Make your movements smooth and flowing. Avoid any fast, jerky motions.

◆ Don't rush through the combinations. Make your moves complete.

◆ Imagine an opponent in front of you if you're working out alone. This will increase your energy level, burn more calories, and improve your workout.

◆ Stay light on your feet. Always be a moving target.

In This Chapter

- ◆ Stepping to success
- ◆ Moving hands, moving feet
- ◆ Combining cardio and toning
- ◆ Coordination drill tips

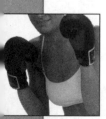 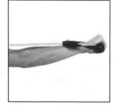 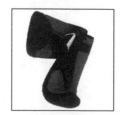 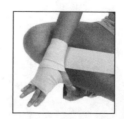 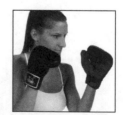 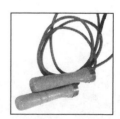

Chapter 17

Getting a Leg Up

The coordination exercises in this chapter are designed to help you move like a real boxer. They'll work your lower body hard, but they'll tone muscle in your upper body, too.

Somewhat similar to a stair-climbing machine, but a lot more fun, these drills combine cardio and toning. Although they can be tough to master, you'll look like a pro when you do. You'll also burn a bunch of calories as you're learning them.

Feet and Hands Together

Coordination drills are similar to trying to rub your tummy and pat your head simultaneously. Moving your arms and legs together in a variety of patterns isn't as easy as just moving around randomly while you throw punches. Coordinating the moves keeps your body guessing. Sometimes you move forward while punching, other times you move backward while kicking. You might Bob and Weave with a Cross while moving forward or Bob and Weave with a Hook while moving backward.

After you master the movements, you'll look and feel like a boxer. Your precise punches and fancy footwork will motivate you to practice more. The longer you practice, the better you'll get, and the more fat you'll lose and muscle you'll tone.

While you're in the learning stage and performing the movements inefficiently, you'll expend a tremendous amount of energy. Because of this, you might catch yourself huffing and puffing as you try to combine your arm and leg movements. Slow down. Pace yourself. Relax and breathe from your diaphragm. Begin slowly and master the form first. You can increase the speed and power of your moves later.

Your brain teaches your body different ways to move, and in doing so increases your movement capabilities. Remember when you learned how to ride a bike? You increased your movement capabilities then, too. Master the exercises in this chapter and you'll be amazed at how coordinated you'll become. Not many people can Bob and Weave with a Right Cross follow up. But you'll be able to.

After you're comfortable with the movements in this chapter, use them as active recovery cycles between your hard effort intervals. For example, after performing 30 seconds of rapid-fire punching, do 30 seconds of Punch Forward, Punch Back until you're ready to perform your next effort interval.

Coordination Drill Tips

These coordination drills are designed to be performed back-to-back in the order they're presented. Do them this way and you'll get an aerobic workout that challenges your mind and body while burning fat and toning muscle.

A great way to begin is to master one part of the movements with your hands first, then feet, or vice versa. As an example, the hand action

for the first two exercises is upward punching. Master it, and then concentrate on the foot movements, which are different for each drill. When you have one movement down fairly well, it's easier to concentrate on the rest.

Keep the following tips in mind as you tackle these drills:

◆ Train in front of a mirror to help check form.

◆ Play your favorite motivational music—whether it's the theme from *Rocky* or Beethoven's *Ninth Symphony*. Let the beat move you around the room.

◆ Keep your upper body relaxed.

◆ Maintain a fighting position at all times—elbows in, hands up, chin down.

◆ Keep your balance by maintaining your center of gravity (shoulders over your hips).

◆ Take small steps forward and backward.

◆ Stay light on the balls of your feet.

◆ Breathe from your diaphragm; that is, breathe from your lower abdomen instead of your upper chest.

The DVD that accompanies this book is a great way to see how to do these drills. Be sure to press "pause" if you need time to gather your thoughts between exercises.

Put these drills together for a great steady state workout. If you want to burn a lot of calories, do them back to back over the course of 30 minutes to 1 hour.

Punch Forward, Punch Back

This is a steady state workout where you perform continuous movement with your large muscle groups just below your anaerobic threshold—the point at which you'll be huffing and puffing. This exercise burns a lot of fat because it takes more energy to punch vertically than it does to punch horizontally. It also increases your coordination because your hands are moving

one way and your feet are moving a different way. You firm up the muscles of your legs and buns at the same time you tone your shoulder and triceps muscles.

Stand facing forward with your arms up in a fighting position. Take small steps forward as you extend your arms up in the air, alternating your punches toward the ceiling. When you reach the front of the room, continue punching while taking small steps backward to your original position.

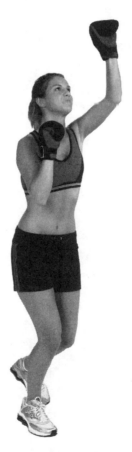

Take small steps and punch straight up into the air.
Keep your back straight, chest out, and eyes up.

Kick Forward, Kick Back

This is another excellent fat burner and coordination drill; however, it can be frustrating until you get your coordination down. Be patient and keep at it.

Punch toward the ceiling as you alternate low kicks forward. Alternate feet and hands—when your right hand is up in the air, your left foot should be out, and vice versa. When you reach the front of the room, continue punching and kicking as you move backward to your original position.

Be careful not to go too fast. If you begin huffing and puffing, slow down and catch your breath.

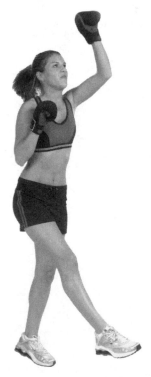

Punch high while throwing low kicks as you step forward. Keep your head up, chest out, and stomach in.

 # Knee Forward, Knee Back

This is an excellent calorie burner that works the muscle on the front of your upper thigh.

Punch toward the ceiling while alternating low knee lifts forward. When you reach the front of the room, reverse your move direction and move backward to your original position as you continue punching and lifting your knees.

Don't try to lift your knees too high—up to your waist or thereabouts is fine. Keep your upper body relaxed throughout this exercise.

 Corner Man

Move purposefully through these stepping drills. Don't just go through the motions. Moving purposefully will help you activate more muscle fibers and will result in a better workout.

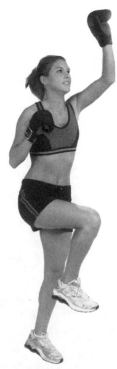

Alternate punches toward the ceiling. Maintain correct posture as you alternate knee lifts.

Boxer's Shuffle Across the Room

The Boxer's Shuffle, which you learned in Chapter 2, is the foundation for all your footwork drills. The Boxer's Shuffle Across the Room activates your calf muscles, thighs, buns, and hamstrings.

Step forward a few inches with your left foot and move your right foot to replace the position of your left foot. Push off with your right foot as you step forward with your left. Continue moving forward in this fashion until you reach the front of the room.

After you reach the front of the room, take an initial step with your right foot while your left foot replaces the position of your right foot.

Push off with your left foot as you step backward with your right foot. Continue moving backward until you reach your original position.

As you get good at this drill, increase the speed of your shuffle. The faster you shuffle, the more calories you burn, and the more fat you lose.

Maintain correct posture with your hands in a fighting position and your upper body relaxed. Try to keep your head and shoulders level when you shuffle. Check your form in the mirror.

Corner Man

The Boxer's Shuffle is the foundation for all footwork drills, so get used to practicing it often. You'll know when you're doing it enough when it invades your dreams!

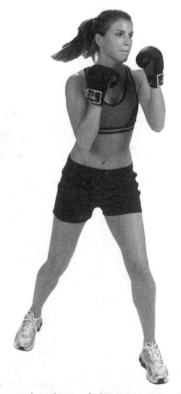

Keep your hands in a fighting position and your upper body relaxed. Stay light on the balls of your feet and keep your shoulders parallel to the floor.

Bob and Weave Forward with Cross

Bob and Weave Forward with Cross will seem impossible unless you follow the direction of the models on the DVD.

Step forward with your left foot and complete a Bob and Weave. On the upward movement, execute a Right Cross to the head of your imaginary opponent.

Imagine you're evading your opponent's punch and follow up with a powerful Right Cross. Keep moving forward, taking small steps, until you reach the front of the room. Move at your own rhythm. Move as slow as you need to maintain proper form.

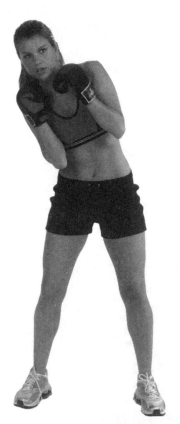

Keep your hands up in a fighting position and your upper body relaxed. Use a Boxer's Shuffle as you step forward across the room.

 # Bob and Weave Backward with Hook

This exercise trains all the muscles in your upper and lower body and is a superior fat-burning move.

Take a step backward with your right foot as you bend at your knees and hips ducking under an imaginary cross. On the upward movement, execute a Left Hook.

Your lower body does the Boxer's Shuffle and your upper body bobs and weaves. At the completion of your Bob and Weave, throw a Left Hook. This exercise is meant to get you from the front of the room to the back of the room.

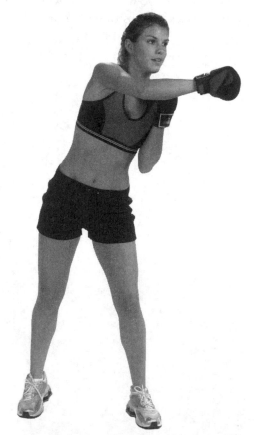

Maintain your upper body in a relaxed fighting position. Move back by bobbing and weaving in a Boxer's Shuffle and complete each movement with a hook.

Jabs Across the Room

This is a great way to practice your jab and footwork and burn calories at the same time.

Take small steps forward with your left foot and throw left jabs until you reach the front of the room. To get back to your original position, take small steps back with your right foot and throw left jabs as soon as your feet are set.

Use the Boxer's Shuffle to cover distance both forward and backward. Be sure to set your feet before you complete each jab. Relax between each move. Exhale at the completion of each jab and contract your abdominal muscles.

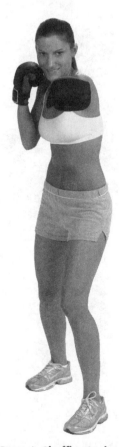

Step using a Boxer's Shuffle. At the completion of each step, throw a Left Jab while maintaining correct posture.

Crosses Across the Room

Crosses Across the Room is an excellent cardio-vascular workout that burns fat and tones muscle.

Step forward with your left foot and as soon as your feet are set, throw a Right Cross. Continue until you reach the front of the room. To get back to your original position, take a step back with your right foot, and when your feet are set, throw a Right Cross.

Use the Boxer's Shuffle to cover the distance and be sure to pivot on your right foot when you begin your cross. Exhale on each punch as you contract your abs.

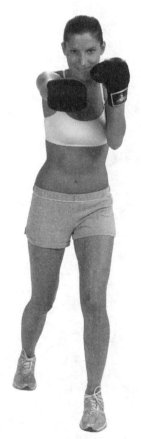

Maintain correct posture as you step forward with your left foot and pivot your right foot into a powerful Right Cross.

Hooks Across the Room

Step forward with your left foot and throw a hook. Continue until you reach the front of the room. To return to your original position, take a step with your right foot and slide your left foot back and execute a Left Hook. Continue until you reach your original position.

Use the Boxer's Shuffle to cover distance and try to stay level so that your head and shoulders are not bobbing up and down with each step.

Begin slowly at first. After you've learned the form, you may move faster to burn additional calories.

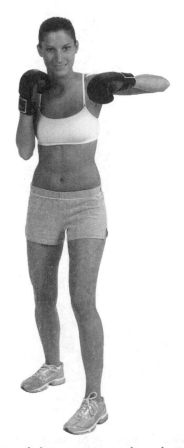

Maintain a fighting position and use the Boxer's Shuffle to step forward and back. Immediately upon completing the step, execute a Left Hook.

Uppercuts Across the Room

Uppercuts Across the Room is an excellent bun, hamstring, and thigh toner.

Walk forward, throwing left and right uppercuts with each step. When you reach the front of the room, reverse your direction and walk backward. Continue throwing uppercuts on each step.

Keep your hands up between uppercuts. Resist the temptation to drop your hands.

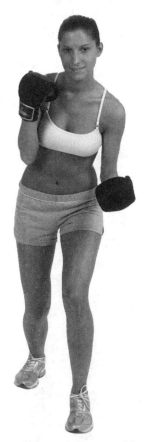

Bend from your knees and hips and keep your back straight. Keep your arms bent at a 90-degree angle at all times.

Corner Man

When you do Uppercuts Across the Room, bend from your knees and hips and then explode like a big spring. Think of your arm as an attachment to your body; it doesn't move on its own.

The Least You Need to Know

◆ Learning to move your hands and feet in different ways and at different angles at the same time is challenging. The mental effort alone burns a few extra calories and improves your motor control, or ability to control your body's movements.

◆ If you have trouble with these drills, concentrate on your hands. After you master your hand movements, concentrate on your feet.

◆ Learn the form first, and then add speed and power. After you feel confident in your form, throw your punches with a little more speed.

◆ Stay just below the level of heavy breathing on these drills. If you start huffing and puffing and burning, you have crossed your anaerobic threshold. Back off. Stay below the burn and you will last longer and burn more fat.

In This Part

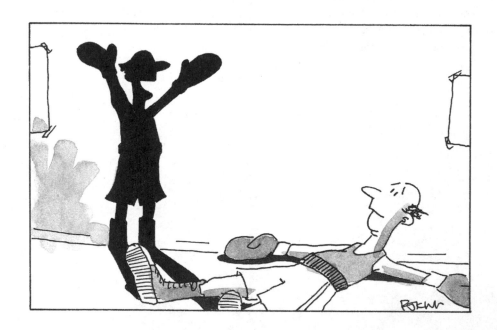

Going the Distance

By now you realize that fitness boxing can be as much a part of your life as brushing your teeth. Fitness boxing is fun, and the benefits go far beyond cosmetic. You feel better and more energized than ever before. Unlike a quick-fix diet or exercise plan, you build your body from the inside out—and the fitness results are lasting.

Part 4 begins with teaching you one of your best tools for getting and staying in shape. Shadowboxing can be performed anywhere whether you are "dressed out" or not. You'll also learn detailed partner workouts that increase the intensity of your program. And before you shower, enjoy the benefits of a boxer's cool down and stretch.

In This Chapter

- Gearing yourself up mentally
- What's involved in a shadowboxing workout
- Training with bodyweight
- The best shadowboxing routines

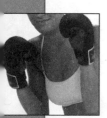
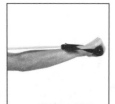
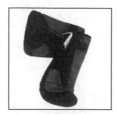
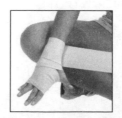
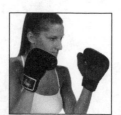
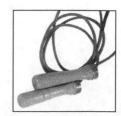

Chapter 18

Solo Workouts: Shadowboxing and Bagwork

If you enjoy working out with others, you might think training alone is the epitome of boredom. But shadowboxing and bagwork are anything but boring. Both offer a great workout during which you can let your imagination run wild. You can throw your punches and duck jabs against the best of them. Before you know it, your workout is over and there are puddles of sweat all around you.

Feeling the need to take out some pent-up aggression? These are the workouts where you can do just about anything you want—within reason, of course!—and there's no harm done.

Exercise and the Mind

Shadowboxing and bagwork require a certain mental focus that training with other people doesn't. You're putting your mind into your muscle and throwing all your basic punches and moves against an imaginary opponent. Every time you throw a punch it scores. You win every time you step into your imaginary ring.

But the keyword here is you. You have to decide how hard you want to work, and without others around you, you might find the going difficult, especially when you start to get tired or when discomfort sets in. It takes mental discipline and perseverance to work out by yourself. But you can do it. Here's how.

Self Talk

Your mind prepares your body for your fitness boxing workout. Your mind also tells your body when to quit. Nerves send messages of discomfort to the spinal cord, which delivers them to your brain.

Instead of focusing on being uncomfortable, use keywords and imagery to reinterpret these signals more positively. Discomfort goes away when you call it something else.

Talk to yourself nicely. Use positive affirmations such as the following:

- ◆ "Shadowboxing makes me stronger."
- ◆ "Every punch I throw gets me one step closer to my goals."
- ◆ "I'm sleek, strong, and beautiful."
- ◆ "The burn in my shoulders is a signal that my muscles are getting firm and toned."

These self-reflections get you pumped up for your workout, help you change your perspective about your body, and help you look at the discomfort of a great workout as enjoyable.

Corner Man

Quitting is usually the first option when confronted with the fatigue and discomfort of a shadowboxing workout; especially if you're training by yourself and there's no accountability. Persevere! You will be glad you did—the benefits of completing these workouts are worth it.

Concentration

Concentrating on what you're doing will put you in control of your workout. Try this: focus exclusively on your jab. Recruit every muscle fiber in your triceps to push through the jab. Choose to feel every aspect of your jab. Visualize fibers splitting and blood pumping to your shoulders, chest, back, and arms.

Or instead of thinking about what you're doing, you can dissociate from the boredom of a tedious drill by setting your mind apart from your body. Focus on the beat of the music and your workout will be over before you know it.

A Little Mind Control

Have the confidence and the expectation that you will get through your shadowboxing workout. Remind yourself that following your effort interval, you get to enjoy a 1-minute, well-deserved recovery.

Teach your body to handle discomfort a little at a time. Reach deep inside and ask yourself to keep going until the end of the round. Don't stop until you hear the "ding" of your timer.

Plan your shadowboxing moves before you do them. Picture yourself performing a perfect jab. When you do, you're sending nervous impulses down the proper neuromuscular pathways. This in itself stimulates muscle fibers and enhances your speed and performance.

Anatomy of a Shadowboxing Workout

A shadowboxing workout consists of a warm up, several rounds of shadowboxing and/or bagwork, and a cool down. In this chapter, you perform the Plank, Torso Toner, and Cross Pivot as your warm up. The Plank strengthens your core. The Torso Toner warms up and firms your waist and back. The Cross Pivot is a total body exercise that reduces body fat and increases muscle tone.

You can shadowbox as a workout in itself, or, if you own a bag, you can use your shadowboxing skills on it.

Bodyweight Warm Ups

Bodyweight moves, which, as the name suggests, call for moving your body against gravity, are a natural outgrowth of shadowboxing. Years ago, boxers didn't lift weights for fear of becoming bulky and slow. Yet they grew sinewy, strong muscles anyway. How? Besides hitting the bag, jumping rope, sparring, and running, they did body weight moves such as the ones in this chapter.

Moves such as the Torso Toner, which also improve core strength and muscular endurance, are convenient and effective and continue today in boxing gyms across the country. They also improve strength, power, speed, and endurance without elaborate training equipment, which makes them great for at-home workouts. By simply bringing your hands a little closer on the Plank or changing the angle that you move on the Torso Toner exercise, you can change the angle of the exercise and work your muscles in a slightly different way.

The following moves provide a good warm up and work various muscle groups at the same time. If you begin to lose your form, stop the exercise. If your back sags or your legs get tired, take a break. Come back when you're revitalized and try it again.

Boxer's Plank

The Plank trains all muscle groups in your body, with particular attention given to the core muscles of the abs and back.

Use the back-straight military push-up position (from your knees or feet) on each set.

Be sure to keep your elbows and knees slightly bent. Breathe normally from your diaphragm. Keep your hands in line with your shoulders and don't let your back sag. If you begin to lose your form, stop the exercise immediately.

If the Plank is too challenging from your feet, try it from your knees.

Begin by doing the Boxer's Plank once and holding it for 3 seconds. Add two sets—that is, do the move twice, holding each time for 3 seconds—per week until you can perform 10 of them.

When you can perform the Plank while maintaining correct form, vary the angle of the exercise to recruit more muscle fibers.

Corner Man

Many strength and conditioning "gurus" argue that bodyweight exercises such as the Plank are ineffective because there is no movement. But this isn't true, as the Plank has been shown to be one of the best exercises for firming and toning the abs and back.

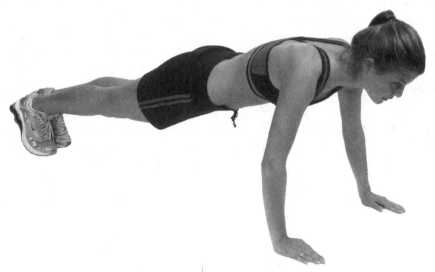

Hold a push-up position with your neck relaxed. Concentrate on contracting the muscles in your abs and back.

Standing Torso Toner, All Directions

The Standing Torso Toner is a core-building move that trains the entire lower torso.

Stand in a fighting stance and imagine an opponent throwing jabs at your head. Slip the imaginary jab in all directions by tilting from your waist. Your movements should be very small and subtle. Be careful that you don't twist or bend too fast or too far.

At first, be very methodical about practicing this exercise. Bend forward, backward, then to your left, finally to your right. Eventually mix up the angles and directions so that you can move spontaneously in any direction.

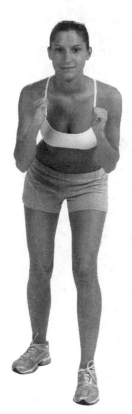

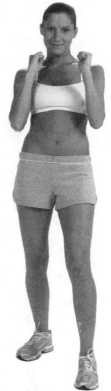

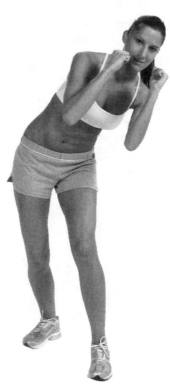

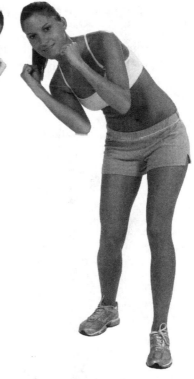

With your hands in a fighting position, lean slightly forward, flexing your spine. Always keep your knees slightly bent. Your upper body should remain relaxed.

Lean slightly backward extending your spine. Move no more than 3 inches. Keep a stable base of support with both knees bent.

Lean a couple inches to your left. Try not to drop your hands and be careful not to lean too far.

Lean a couple inches to your right. Keep your head in line with your body and breathe from your diaphragm.

Cross Pivot to Power Your Punch

The Cross Pivot is a great way to power your core. When you pivot your foot and shift your hips, your abs naturally twist and contract. This not only improves the power in your Right Cross, but it strengthens the muscles in your thighs, buns, hamstrings, abs, and back for a firm, powerful look.

Begin in a fighting stance with both feet pointing at a 45-degree angle. Bend your knees over your toes and keep your weight evenly distributed.

Contract your abdominal muscles as you simultaneously pivot on the ball of your right foot so that your right heel is off the floor. Your left knee remains bent while your right leg straightens slightly, keeping your knee soft. Pivot back into a fighting stance and repeat. Move slowly at first, so your feet, knees, and hips are in alignment.

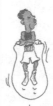

Sweet Science

Twisting of the body has been named the "serape effect" in exercise physiology research terms because of the powerful muscular forces created by the hip and torso twist.

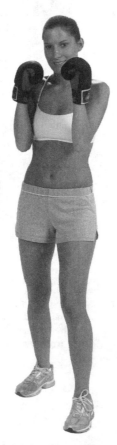

Begin in a fighting position with your upper body relaxed and your back straight.

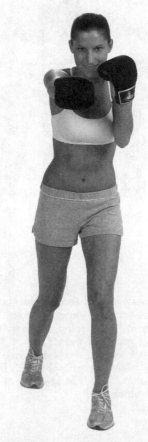

Keep your hands up as you pivot your right foot. This begins the power chain that travels through your thighs, buns, back, and abs. Exhale through pursed lips as you complete the exercise.

"Ding": Start Your Workout

Some of the following routines are straight shadowboxing, some incorporate bags. Be creative. Do different drills on different days. Rather than working on the same punches day in and day out, vary your routine so your mind and body stay fresh.

Just as you can walk, jog, or run, you can shadowbox as hard or as easy as you want to. You can do a sweat-free shadowboxing exercise for 3 minutes during your coffee break at work, or a 30-minute, high-intensity shadowboxing workout as prescribed in the following section—it's your choice.

If you dislike a drill, substitute another in its place. Enjoy your entire workout or you will find excuses not to train.

Work on your weaknesses and maintain your strengths. Spend a few extra minutes each day working on the boxing skills that you need to improve.

If possible, shadowbox in front of a mirror so you can check your techniques and perfect your form.

Knockout Punch

Never do two hard bag workout days in a row. That would be the same as training your chest hard in the weight room for two consecutive days. It's much better to take a day off between hard workouts.

Sample Boxer's Workout #1: The Battle Begins

This 30-minute, high-intensity shadowboxing workout involves 3-minute work cycles interspersed with 1-minute active recovery periods of walking in place. Shadowboxing is followed by simulated sparring, focus mitt training, and finally bagwork.

Warm up with jumping jack punches or footwork drills—5 minutes.

Do upper body shoulder and torso stretches—3 minutes.

Do three 3-minute rounds of shadowboxing with a 1-minute rest between each round. Your first round is going through the motions of all your punches. Your second round consists of punches, slips, and bobbing and weaving at a medium intensity. Your third round is high-intensity shadowboxing against an imaginary opponent. Timed 3-minute rounds are the heart of your workout.

Power training is next. Three rounds on the heavy bag is all you need to round out a great workout. Practice all your favorite combinations.

Cool down with 5 minutes of core training and another 5 minutes of stretching.

Sample Boxer's Workout #2: Mixing It Up

This 18-minute workout is good if you're a little short on time. Don't rest between workout segments beyond the time it takes to move from one exercise to the next.

Jog in Place—1 minute.

Jumping Jacks—2 minutes.

Jump Rope—3 minutes.

Shadowbox—3 minutes. Throw all your punches, and use all your defensive maneuvers. Work in front of a mirror to check your form.

Boxer's Shuffle—1 minute.

Heavy bag—3 minutes. Work on your jab, cross, hook, and uppercut, then throw combinations.

Bob and Weave—1 minute.

Heavy bag—3 minutes. Perform these combinations in sequence without rest between sets: 1-1, 1-1-1, 1-2, 1-2-3, 1-2-3-4. (1 = jab, 2 = cross, 3 = hook, 4 = uppercut).

Cool down and stretch—1 minute.

Sample Boxer's Workout #3: Rapid Fire

Rapid Fire is a string of all-out punches thrown consecutively for ten 30-second intervals—kind of like sprinting with your arms. They are quick, high-intensity workouts that will improve your short-term endurance as well as your speed and power.

You'll need a bag for these workouts. They are physically demanding so be mentally prepared to give your best effort.

After your 5-minute shadowboxing warm up, do 10 rounds of 30-second Rapid Fire 1, 2 punches with 30 seconds rest between rounds.

Sample Boxer's Workout #4: Power Workout

This drill develops strength and power. Be sure to wear hand wraps, as each punch you throw will be at maximum power.

Throw crosses, hooks, and uppercuts with your entire body behind each punch. Keep your hands up in a fighting position and move around the bag as if it was an opponent.

Ten 60-second rounds with 30 seconds rest between rounds is plenty.

Sample Boxer's Workout #5: Putting It All Together

This bag workout puts everything together—basic punches, Power Punching, and Rapid Fire drills.

Begin with precision punching while you're fresh. Proceed to power drills, and finish with conditioning drills. Allow a 1-minute rest between each round.

Warm up shadowboxing—2 minutes.

Perform three 3-minute rounds with a 1-minute rest between each round. Focus on precision. This is the time to perfect your form. Use multiple combinations. Move right to left and then left to right. Keep your hands up and use Slips, and Bob and Weave.

Do three 30-second rounds of power punching. Go at maximum power with an emphasis on full-out, hitting-through-the-bag punches.

Perform five 30-second Rapid Fire sets. Each set consists of 1, 2 punches thrown as fast as you can with maximum speed.

Cool down and stretch—5 minutes.

The Least You Need to Know

◆ Shadowboxing and bagwork are great solo exercises that are anything but boring.

◆ Be creative. Do different drills on different days. Vary your routine so your mind and body stay fresh.

◆ If you dislike a drill, substitute another in its place. Enjoy your entire workout or you will find excuses not to train.

◆ Never do two hard bag workout days in a row. Take a day off between hard workouts. You want your body to recover from these heavy workouts.

◆ If you begin losing form, stop the exercise. Take a quick rest and try it again when you're revitalized.

In This Chapter

- ◆ The benefits of partner drill workouts
- ◆ Training tips for partner drills
- ◆ Fun drills to do with a partner
- ◆ Working with focus mitts

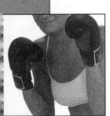 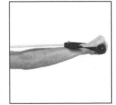 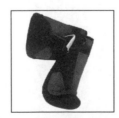 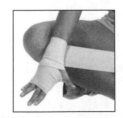 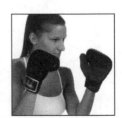 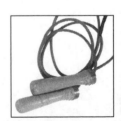

Chapter 19

Partner Drills

Want to get a taste for what it's like to go a few rounds in the ring? Rustle up a partner and do some partner training drills! Not only can partner training drills simulate situations you'd actually face in the ring, it's fantastic for motivation and calorie burning, too.

This chapter gives you some suggestions for training drills that will increase your strength, balance, and muscular endurance, and that will also give you a feel for what being in the ring is all about.

What Partner Drills Do for You

Practically every workout in this book can be done with a partner. There are no programs that are set in stone and that can't be modified. Some are even better when you have someone else alongside you going through the same paces you are. That said, there are some, such as the focus mitt routines in this chapter, that you can't do on your own and you definitely need a partner for.

Timing is the ability to see an action and react to it, and it's an important component to boxing and to fitness boxing. Timing is also something that training with a partner is good for, too. You learn timing through sparring and partner drills. You can't learn it by hitting the heavy bag or by shadowboxing, as you really need to have someone in front of you either working drills or really trying to hit you. Only by constantly seeing punches coming at you will you be able to beat your opponent to the punch.

Knockout Punch

Partner training is fun, but be especially vigilant to prevent a needless injury. Hold the pads properly, be sure your partner knows what technique you are preparing to perform, and allow your partner to move at his or her own pace, not yours. Be sensitive about how your partner is feeling and adjust the movements accordingly throughout the workout.

Getting the Most Out of Partner Drills

One of the best benefits of partner drill training is the synergy that develops when you encourage your partner and vice versa. It helps both you and your partner stay excited and pumped up during training.

There are many different ways to structure your partner drill program—it all depends on your preferences and the equipment you have at hand. That said, there are some general tips for partner drills that are good to keep in mind:

◆ Be sure your partner knows exactly what drill you're performing—no guessing. Eliminate chances for accidents by knowing your partner's agenda.

◆ If you're using focus mitts, be careful to just touch the mitts. Don't hit through them, as doing so could injure your partner.

◆ Plan your drills so you and your partner get equal workout time.

◆ Incorporate drills at varying intensities, especially if you and your partner are at different fitness levels.

◆ Take frequent breaks between high-intensity drills. When it's your turn to hold the pads, consider that a break. While your partner is working you are resting and vice-versa.

Finger Drill

This great drill will help improve the speed of your reaction time. Stand facing your partner with your hands up and your index fingers pointed up. Your partner faces you in a fighting stance. When you drop your right finger, your partner throws a jab. When you drop your left finger, your partner throws a cross. Continue this drill performing five repetitions with each hand for a total of 10 reps. Switch roles and repeat.

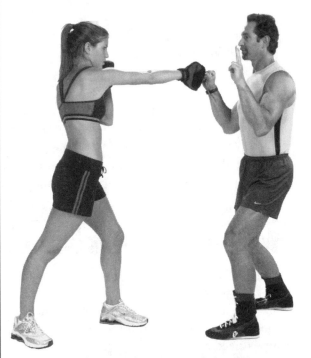

Relax with correct posture in a fighting position. Bounce lightly on the balls of your feet. React as quickly as you can when your partner drops her finger.

Front Back Side-to-Side Drill

This vigorous drill burns fat, tones lower body muscles, and strengthens your core.

Stand facing your partner with your right arm up. Your partner is facing you in a fighting stance. When you move your hand forward, your partner shuffles back. When you move your hand back, your partner shuffles forward. When you move your hand to the right, your partner shuffles to her left. When you move your hand to the left, your partner shuffles to the right. Continue moving forward, back, and side to side for 10 movement repetitions. Switch roles and repeat.

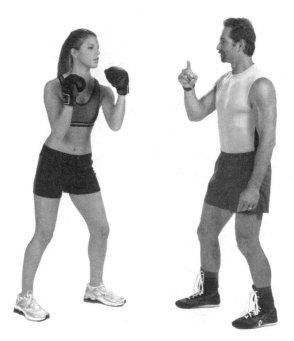

Maintain correct posture in a fighting position. Bounce lightly on the balls of your feet. React as quickly as you can to your partner's directions.

Follow the Leader Drill

Face your partner with both of you in fighting stances. When you throw a jab, cross, hook, or uppercut, your partner tries to mimic you and beat you to the punch. Switch roles and repeat.

Corner Man

Any time you perform a reaction time drill such as Follow the Leader, you may feel an adrenaline surge that increases your energy expenditure. Your body is in fight-or-flight mode and is ready for action. Capitalize on this rush of energy by picking up the pace.

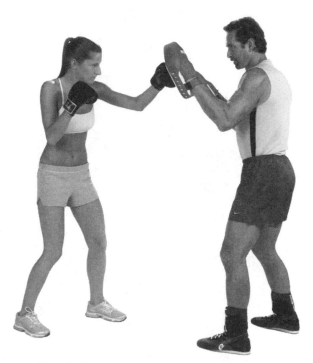

Stand in a fighting stance and react to your partner's cues as quickly as you can.

Counter a Jab Drill

This exercise is a fun way to tone up the muscles in the sides of your waist.

You and your partner face each other in a fighting stance. She slowly throws a jab toward your face. Slip her jab to the right, then to the left. Continue slipping the jab for 10 reps, then switch roles and repeat.

When you slip the jab, tilt your upper body by slightly bending your knees. Keep your head and neck in line with your body. Imagine that your neck is bolted onto your shoulders.

Be careful to move very slowly throughout the entire drill.

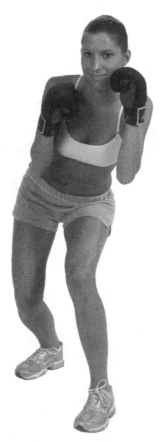

Keep your upper body relaxed and your hands up. When you slip the jab, be sure not to drop your hands.

Counter a Cross Drill

The Bob and Weave portion of the Counter a Cross drill tones your buns, hips, and thighs and it's a great fat burner.

You and your partner face each other in a fighting stance. Throw a slow cross toward your partner's head. Allow her time to react by executing a Bob and Weave and then counter with a Right Cross. Continue for 10 repetitions. Switch roles and repeat.

Move very slowly through this drill. Be sure to give your partner plenty of time to react.

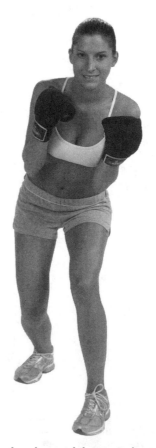

Keep your hands up while you Bob and Weave. When you throw a Right Cross, use your momentum from the Bob and Weave to power your punch.

Partner Drills with Focus Mitts

Most people find focus mitt training the favorite part of their partner drill workouts. You get to hit something, you burn calories, and the "fun" component is built-in.

Have your partner hold the focus mitts in front of her shoulders with her elbows bent at a 90-degree angle. Arms should be relaxed. Whenever you throw a punch, it should always be across your body. As examples:

◆ If your partner holds out her right hand, you'll throw a Right Cross.

◆ If she holds her left hand out, you'll throw a Left Jab.

◆ If the left mitt is at eye level, turned out so that the pad is facing inward, try a Left Hook.

◆ If the right mitt is at head level, pad facing down, use a Right Uppercut.

Knockout Punch

Make contact with the pad and retract your arm as quickly as you can back to a fighting position. Touch the pad, never hit through it. If you try to hit through the pad, you may injure your partner.

 Jab

Begin in a fighting stance and step into a Left Jab. Extend your arm keeping your elbow close to your body for as long as possible. Touch the pad with the first two knuckles of your hand. Retract your arm as fast as you extended it back to your fighting position. Continue for 10 repetitions.

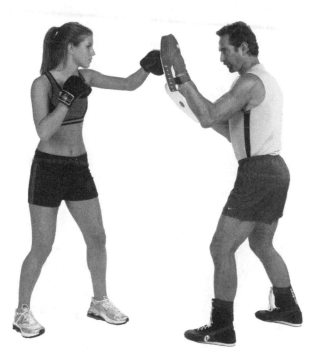

Begin in a relaxed fighting position. As you continue to extend your fist toward the target, keep your right hand up and exhale through pursed lips.

Right Cross

The power in your Right Cross comes from your body, not your arm. Begin the power chain by pivoting on the ball of your right foot. Allow the power to flow through your body until it leaves your fist and makes contact with the pad. Instead of pushing the pad, pop it. Pop the pad without following through. Bring your arm back into a fighting position as quickly as you can.

You'll hear a "popping" sound when you throw a perfect cross. Continue for 10 repetitions.

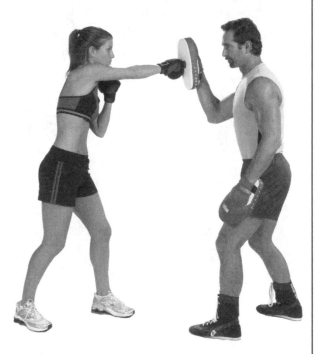

Relax in a fighting stance and without retracting your right hand, move it straight toward the target. Just before your right hand hits the target, complete your exhalation and contract your abs. Keep your left hand up the entire time.

Hook

The Left Hook is the only punch where you bring your forearm up parallel to the floor. All the other punches are initiated keeping the elbows in close to the body. For this reason, the hook utilizes different muscles in your chest and shoulders.

Begin in a fighting stance. As soon as you begin your left foot pivot, bring your arm up so that by the time you complete your pivot, you can follow through with your punch. Continue for 10 repetitions.

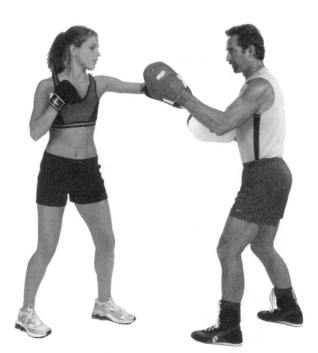

Begin from a fighting stance with your whole body relaxed. Raise your arm and keep your elbow bent at 90 degrees as you pivot your left foot inward. Just before your first two knuckles hit the target, exhale through pursed lips and contract your abs.

Uppercut

The uppercut is a full-body workout toning your thighs, buns, hamstrings, and abs. It's a power punch that gets its energy from the legs.

Begin in a fighting stance. Drop your shoulder so that your elbow slides by your hip as your knees bend. Extend your knees and exhale through pursed lips as you hit the pad with your first two knuckles. Continue for 10 repetitions.

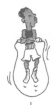
Sweet Science

Most of the uppercut's power comes from extending the knees from a half-squat position.

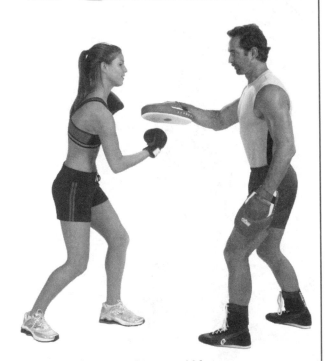

Bend from your knees and lift up into your punch. Keep your elbows bent at 90 degrees. When you follow through, your arm remains at a 90-degree angle.

 ## Duck Under

Doing Duck Under reps is similar to doing squats in the weight room except the fun factor is ten-fold. You tone your thighs, buns, and hamstrings while you improve your reaction time and confidence.

Duck as your partner sweeps her right arm slowly toward your head. Your upper body remains in a fighting stance throughout the Duck Under. Bend your knees and keep your eyes on your partner. Be sure to keep your back straight and your eyes up. Keep your eyes on your partner the entire time. Keep your hands up and exhale as you duck.

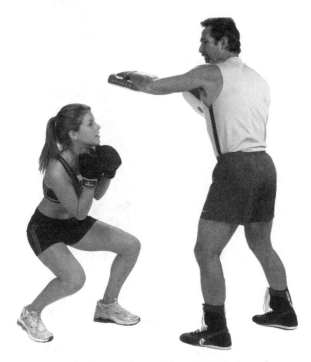

Keep your back straight and time your duck so that your partner's pad misses your head by at least a foot.

Duck Under and Counter Punch

This drill puts it all together. You train your thighs, buns, and hamstrings by bending into a squat. Then when you use your Right Cross to Counter Punch, you twist the rest of your body into your effort, making for a great full-body exercise. Defending and attacking delivers an adrenaline rush.

Duck as your partner sweeps her right arm slowly toward your head. Be sure to keep your back straight and your eyes up. Then as you extend your knees back into your fighting position, throw a Right Cross Counter Punch toward the focus mitt that your partner is holding in her left hand.

Be alert in your fighting stance as you wait for your partner to attack with the pad. As soon as she moves her arm, duck under it keeping your hands in a fighting position.

Do this exercise very slowly until you get the hang of it.

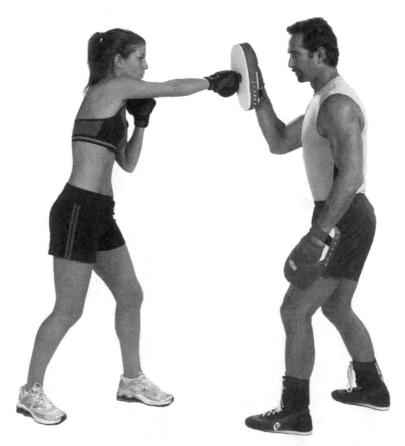

As soon as you have successfully evaded the attack, throw your Right Cross Counter Punch to the opposite focus mitt.

The Least You Need to Know

◆ Be sure your partner knows exactly what drill you're performing. Eliminate chances for accidents by knowing your partner's agenda, too. Go slow and steady to prevent injuries to you and your partner.

◆ Encourage your partner and she will encourage you. Stay excited and pumped up during your training and your partner will be more likely to do the same.

◆ Nothing beats partner focus mitt training for motivation and calorie burning. You get to punch at focus mitts at all different angles and re-create situations that would actually occur in the ring.

◆ Be careful not to hit through the focus mitts, just touch them. Hitting through the mitt can injure your partner.

In This Chapter

- ◆ Cooling it down
- ◆ Stretching it out
- ◆ Dynamic stretching
- ◆ Stretching do's and don'ts

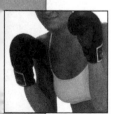
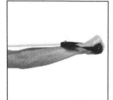
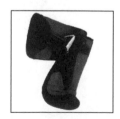
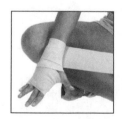
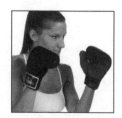
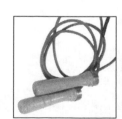

Chapter **20**

The Final Round

A good cool down is always important after any kind of workout, but it's especially so after high-intensity exercise such as fitness boxing.

Like warming up, there's a right way and a wrong way to cool down. This chapter shows you how.

Cooling Things Down

Not only does a proper cool down gradually return your heart rate and blood pressure to normal after exercise, it also helps remove lactic acid build-up in the bloodstream and muscles and will make you feel better after your workout. Walking in place or shadowboxing in slow motion circulates your blood to remove waste products and make you feel better.

Cooling down properly will also help your muscles convert the lactate they produced during your workout into glycogen. Glycogen is the storage form of energy in your muscles. If you cool down properly, you should feel great after your workout because your muscles are returning to their before-workout state.

Cooling down after a workout also prevents feeling lightheaded, which can happen if you stop your exercise too quickly, especially at high-intensity levels.

Cooling down allows blood to circulate throughout your body instead of pooling in your legs. If you don't cool down, your brain might not receive the blood it needs, which leads to that dizzy feeling.

Knockout Punch

Muscular soreness felt a few days after a workout is a result of cellular trauma caused by torn or damaged tissue. Damaged muscle tissue causes inflammation that can hamper you for a few days after your workout, which is why it's important to cool down and stretch after you're done working out.

If you're coming off a hard cardio workout, simply gradually decrease your exertion level until your heart rate approaches your normal resting level. As an example, if you've been doing roadwork, slow to a jog for a few minutes, then to a walk until your heart rate is where it should be.

If you've been lifting hard, finish your routine with a light set or two, lifting very light weights. Follow this with 5 minutes or so of light cardio. If you've been practicing your punches, shadowboxing in slow motion for a few minutes should do the trick. Be sure to keep your legs moving, too.

To cool down correctly, allow your heart rate to drop to somewhere between your resting rate and about 120 beats per minute (bpm). You can measure this by using a heart rate monitor during your workouts. These devices range in price from around $40 to more than $100 and are excellent training tools in general, as they make it easy to keep track of your heart rate and your exertion levels while you're exercising.

If you don't have a heart rate monitor, you can measure your heart rate by taking your pulse at your carotid artery on the side of your neck. Place your index finger and middle finger gently on your carotid artery until you feel your pulse. Count your pulse for 6 seconds and multiply that number by 10 for beats per minute.

You'll know when you've cooled down enough by when your breathing is rhythmic and relaxed with no huffing and puffing. When you get there, it's time to stretch things out.

Corner Man

To determine your resting heart rate (RHR), measure your heart rate the minute you wake up in the morning. Don't use an alarm clock to get you up as it could startle you and send your heart rate zooming before you get out of bed. Do this drill for seven consecutive mornings, then take the average of your readings to get your RHR. You can estimate your maximum heart rate (MHR) with this simple formula: 220 − your age in years.

Stretching Things Out

There are two basic ways to stretch out—*static* and *dynamic*. Dynamic is the more beneficial of the two, as it prevents injury and takes you through the range of motion that you use during fitness boxing.

Clear as a Bell

Static stretching is holding a particular set of muscles in a stretched position for 15 to 30 seconds. **Dynamic stretching** calls for moving through the stretches and extending the muscles through a specific range of motion.

High-level athletes prefer dynamic stretching to passive. Not only do you burn more calories during dynamic stretching, as you're not just holding the stretch, you also move through the same patterns you used during your workout. This improves your coordination, balance, and skill to a much greater extent than static stretching.

Dynamic stretching calls for the following:

◆ Stretching the muscle until you feel tension for 3 seconds

◆ Flexing the same muscle for 3 seconds

◆ Relaxing the muscle

This sequence will allow you to stretch the muscle even farther when you stretch it again.

You can use ropes, brooms, or no equipment at all and still get a great dynamic stretch. Simply move your muscles in the opposite direction that you would move them during flexion.

The dynamic stretches in this chapter should be performed with as many sets as it takes to reach a maximum range of motion in any given direction. Generally three sets of 10 repetitions are plenty.

Corner Man

You can stretch any time during the day, not just after training. When you're at work or in the car, take a few seconds to stretch. Stretch slowly and gradually and not too intensely unless you have a chance to warm up first. You don't need any equipment to get a great stretch.

Always stretch to the point of tension, never pain. Other things to keep in mind for a good stretching routine:

◆ **Go slow.** Speeding through stretches diminishes the pleasure and the benefits.

◆ **Relax.** Exhale through each movement and enjoy it.

◆ **Never stretch a cold muscle.** Always stretch after your workout. Doing so will improve your flexibility and help your muscles recover more fully after your workouts.

Calf Stretch

To stretch your calf muscles (gastrocnemius), assume a lunge position. Keep your back heel on the floor and your back leg almost completely straight as you lean into your front leg. You should feel the stretch in the back of your lower leg.

Contract your calf muscle for 3 seconds by pressing the ball of your foot into the floor. Relax your calf muscle for 3 seconds, then stretch a bit farther.

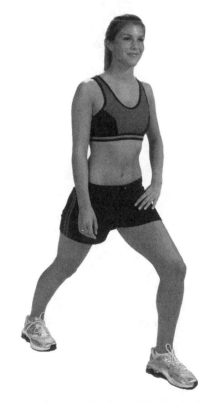

Keep your chest up, back straight, and abs tight. Lean into your stretch and relax. Contract your calf for 3 seconds, then relax again and stretch.

Arms Up Stretch

Spending a lot of time in the Boxer's Crouch keeps you in a flexed, closed position. The Arms Up Stretch opens you up, extends your spine, and feels great.

Hold onto the medicine ball and stand and reach up as high as you can with both arms over your head. Feel the stretch in your upper back. Contract these back muscles for 3 seconds. Relax. Stretch a little higher. Stop when you feel tension. Hold for 3 seconds. Relax.

If you don't have a ball, just reach up as high as you can.

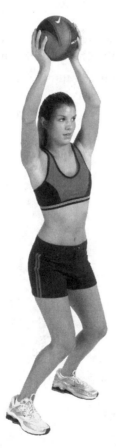

Hold the ball up as high as you can while keeping your upper body relaxed. Maintain correct posture.

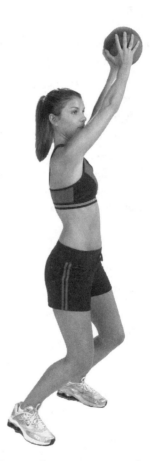

Contract the muscles in your upper back and then relax. See if you can stretch just a bit farther. Hold for 3 seconds, then relax.

Boxing Twist

Boxing Twists stretch out the muscles on the side of your abs called your obliques. It's important to stretch these muscles as most boxing moves require a lot of work out of them.

Hold the ball between your hands. Rotate, turning slowly to the left and then to the right. Start out with the ball close to your body. Do not "suck in," but keep your torso elongated, abs firm.

When you reach the end range of motion on each side, hold for 3 seconds and contract your stomach muscles. Keep your torso stable. Then relax and see if you can stretch a little farther. Hold for 3 seconds. Relax and switch to the other side and repeat the same sequence.

Keep your knees bent and your abs tucked in with your back straight and long.

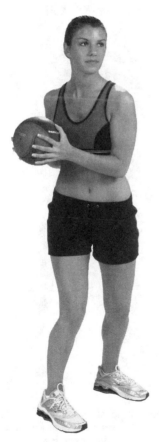

Maintain correct posture and turn slowly until you feel a stretch. Hold for 3 seconds, then stretch a little farther.

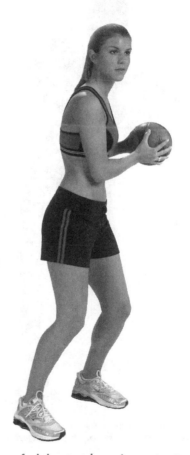

When you feel the stretch again, contract your ab muscles for 3 seconds. Relax, stretch a little farther. Switch sides and repeat.

Bob and Weave Stretch

This is a dynamic stretch using continuous motion that stretches the muscles in your abs, chest, and back. Because you're continually moving through this stretch, you're actively flexing and relaxing muscles which allows you to stretch farther than a normal static stretch where you just hold the position.

Don't stop at any time during this exercise. Each time you perform a repetition, attempt to stretch a little bit farther.

Grab your jump rope in both hands. Position your hands a little more than shoulder-width apart and slip the rope behind your shoulders, keeping it taut. Keep your hands up and elbows in and Bob and Weave to the right. Then Bob and Weave to the left. Continue alternating sides.

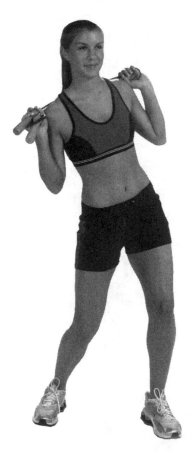

Begin moving in a very small "U" pattern up and down and to the side bobbing and weaving.

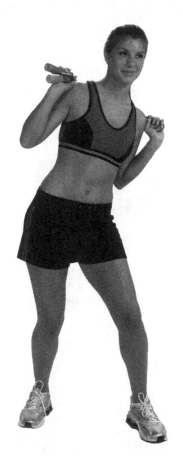

Increase your range of movement so that you begin to feel the stretch on each rep. Relax through the entire exercise.

Neck Stretch

This is a very relaxing stretch and a great way to cool down.

Stand comfortably, and then bring your chin toward your chest. Contract the muscles in the back of your neck. Relax and stretch a bit farther. Then contract the muscles in the front of your neck. Relax and stretch a bit farther. Then bring your right ear toward your right shoulder. Contract the muscles in the right side of your neck. Relax them and stretch a bit farther.

Contract the muscles in the left side of your neck. Relax and stretch toward your right side.

Then bring your left ear toward your left shoulder. Contract the muscles in the left side of your neck. Relax them and stretch a bit farther. Contract the muscles in the right side of your neck. Relax and stretch toward your left side.

Don't try to stretch too far at first. Stop as soon as you feel light tension in any direction.

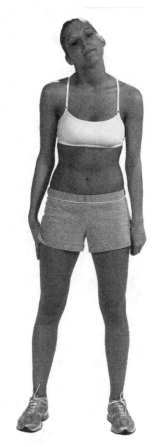

Relax into each stretch. Move slowly and hold each
stretch for 3 seconds.

Boxer Bar

This stretch feels great and helps you discern the specific muscles in your abs that work to power your punches.

Place a broomstick across your shoulders. Stand tall with your feet shoulder-width apart and your arms draped over the stick. Keeping your abs tight, do a tight, small, slow twist to the left and hold for 3 seconds. Then twist to the right and hold for 3 seconds. Exhale each time you twist to the side and inhale as you move back toward the middle.

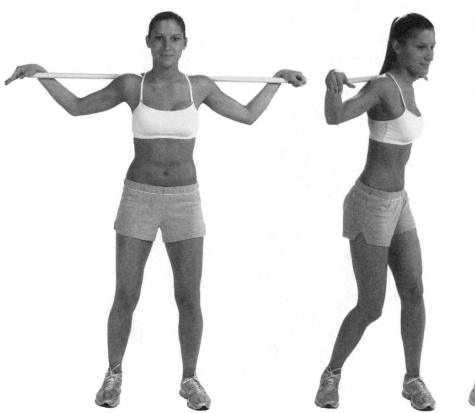

Stand in correct posture with your arms draped over the bar. Keep your knees bent and breathe from your diaphragm.

Try to go a little bit farther each time you twist. When you feel tension, stop, flex, and hold for 3 seconds.

Relax into each stretch and use the bar for leverage so you can hold your stretch more effectively.

Side Twist

Side Twists are a great stretch that you can do any time throughout the day as you don't need any equipment for them. This stretch also reminds you to keep your hands up in the fighting position at all times.

Bring your hands up into a fighting position. Twist from your waist side to side. Move very slowly into each twist. When you feel tension, stop, flex your abs, and then try to move a little farther in that same direction. Hold for 3 seconds. Relax and twist in the other direction and repeat.

As you improve your flexibility, twist farther on each repetition.

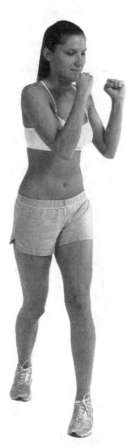

Begin in a fighting position with your knees bent and back straight. Exhale into your twist and hold when you feel tension.

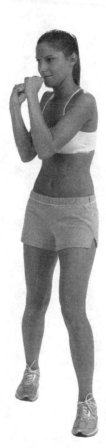

Twist in each direction and make sure your head follows your movement as if it was bolted on your shoulders. Keep your back straight and breathe from your diaphragm.

Shoulder Roll

When you hold your hands up in the fighting position for long periods, your shoulders need a break. The Shoulder Roll feels great and it's a perfect exercise to end your cool down with.

Stand with your feet shoulder-width apart and your upper body tall yet relaxed. Gently roll your shoulders forward. Stop when you feel the stretch. Flex your shoulder muscles for 3 seconds, then relax.

Then roll your shoulders backward. Remember to keep your head up and breathe from your diaphragm.

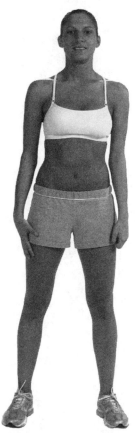

Whether you roll your shoulders forward or backward, keep your head up and breathe from your diaphragm.

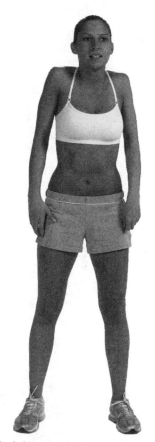

When you feel the stretch, flex the muscles between your shoulder blades and hold for 3 seconds, then relax.

A Final Word

As you have hopefully discovered, an uppercut here and a Bob-and-Weave there can make fitness fun. And if you like what you're doing, you are likely to do more of it. Whether skipping rope or pounding the heavy bag, there can be nothing more satisfying than completing a fitness boxing workout.

This book has been just part of your journey toward fitness, not your destination. You can always get better and fitter, make your jab faster, develop more power in your cross, use more of your body in your hook and uppercut. The byproduct of all of this fun and activity is being in the best shape of your life!

The Least You Need to Know

◆ A good cool down is as important as a good warm up.

◆ Dynamic stretching is better than static stretching. It prevents injury, works your range of motion, and burns calories, too.

◆ Never stretch to the point where you feel pain. Tension is good; pain isn't.

◆ You can stretch any time during the day, not just after training.

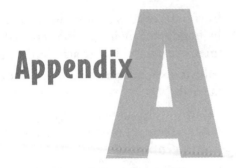

Appendix A

Glossary

abdominals   Flat, band-like muscles that connect the pelvis to the ribcage.

abductors   Outer thigh muscles.

active recovery   Performing some type of moderate activity after a high-intensity move to reduce toxin accumulation after exercise.

adductors   Inner thigh muscles.

aerobic base   Building a strong aerobic base means that you train at a pace where you could carry on a conversation, but if you speed up you will start huffing and puffing.

aerobic exercise   Long duration, low intensity exercise that uses large muscle groups in a rhythmic fashion.

anaerobic exercise   High-intensity, short duration activities.

anaerobic threshold (AT)   The point at which your muscles burn and you begin huffing and puffing. Training just below your AT helps delay the onset of fatigue so you can last long enough to complete your entire fitness boxing program.

arm flexors   Muscles on the front of the upper arm, consisting of the biceps brachii, brachialis, and brachioradialis.

association   Focusing on the activity being performed.

atrophy   Shrinking in size of some part or organ of the body, usually caused by injury, disease, or lack of use.

bag gloves (training gloves)   Padded gloves used to protect the hands when hitting heavy or speed bags.

Basal Metabolic Rate (BMR)   Energy expenditure at rest.

burn   Burning sensation in the muscles caused by buildup of hydrogen ions created through intense exercise. Lactic acid buffers the burn.

caloric expenditure   Amount of calories burned.

calorie   The amount of energy required to raise the temperature of 1 gram of water 1 degree centigrade.

carbohydrates   Fruits, veggies, grains, bread, and pasta are some examples of carbs. They contain carbon, hydrogen, and oxygen and are 4.1 calories per gram.

cardio boxing   *See* fitness boxing.

cardio-kickboxing   An aerobic-anaerobic exercise program using punches, kicks, strikes, and blocks.

cardiovascular system   Made up of the heart, lungs, blood vessels, arteries, and veins.

circuit training   Moving from one exercise to the next with little rest in-between exercises.

compound set   Performing two or more exercises for the same muscle group, such as doing biceps curls followed by reverse curls.

cool-down   Gradual slowing down of movement and heart rate after exercise.

cross   Throwing your right hand straight to the target. Also called a right cross or straight cross.

cross training   Performing two or more types of exercises in a single workout or alternating in successive workouts.

dehydration   The loss of excessive amounts of water and electrolytes from the body.

deltoids   Shoulder muscles, including the anterior deltoid, medial deltoid, and posterior deltoid.

diaphragm   A flat layer of muscle that separates the chest from the abdomen.

dissociation   Focusing on something other than the activity at hand.

Duck Under   Bending the knees to evade a punch to the head.

duration   Workout length.

dynamic stretching   Using one's own muscle power to stretch the limbs through a range of motion.

endorphins   Natural, morphine-like substances produced in the body in response to pain, exercise, or the pain of exercise.

erector spinae   A long muscle mass that extends down the back. It connects the pelvis and the ribcage to the spine.

exercise intensity   How hard you work out.

external obliques   Muscles on the sides of the stomach.

fast-twitch muscle fibers   Large muscle fibers that respond to high-intensity training.

fiber   The indigestible form of carbohydrate found in plant foods.

fitness boxing (cardio boxing)   A workout that combines traditional boxing moves and training approaches with modern cardiovascular and muscle-conditioning methods.

free weights   Weights that are not attached to a machine and can be freely moved.

frequency   The number of times that something happens during a particular period of time, such as how many times a week someone works out.

gastrocnemius   The long, sleek muscle on the lower leg.

gluteal muscles   The three muscles of the upper thigh and hip that are the largest muscle group in the body. They consist of the gluteus maximus, minimus, and medius.

glycemic index   A measure of how quickly food enters your bloodstream from your digestive system.

hamstrings The muscles on the back of the upper leg, consisting of the semitendinosis, semimembranosis, and biceps femoris.

hand wraps A pair of cloth strips resembling an ace bandage used to protect the wrist and knuckles when hitting a heavy bag.

heavy bag A bag filled with hard or soft material used for punching or kicking. Also called a punching bag.

iliopsoas muscles The two muscles located on either side of the lumbar vertebrae that are used to lift the knees.

imagery A psychological strategy designed to help improve physical performance.

internal obliques The abdominal muscles under the external obliques.

interval training Periods of high-intensity movement followed by recovery segments put together into effort-recovery cycles.

intervertebral disk Small, energy-absorbing, sponge-like cushions located between the vertebrae of the spine.

jab A straight punch.

lactate threshold When the muscles produce more lactate than they can clear out.

lactic acid A byproduct of the incomplete breakdown of carbohydrates during anaerobic exercise.

latissimus dorsi The large "V"-shaped muscle of the upper back. Often referred to as "lats."

left hook A left-handed roundhouse punch.

ligament Fibrous connective tissue that holds bone to cartilage, bone to bone, and supports the joints.

lumbar spine The five lower vertebrae of the spine.

lunge An exercise used to tone the quadriceps, gluteals, and hamstrings.

medicine ball Also known as a power ball, a small ball weighing between four and eight pounds and generally about five inches in diameter, used to improve power.

mitts (focus mitts) Target pads used by boxing trainers that are about 5 inches long and 2 inches wide. The trainer holds the mitts and the boxer punches at them at different speeds and angles.

muscle confusion Changing your workout program so that your muscles don't adapt to your exercise routine.

muscle metabolism Synonymous with the energy production of your muscle. The more muscle you have on your body, the higher your metabolism.

parasympathetic nervous system One of the two branches of the autonomic nervous system. It helps to regulate digestion, circulation, voiding, and other bodily functions. It acts to slow bodily functions.

pectorals The chest muscles, consisting of the pectoralis major and pectoralis minor.

plyometrics Power drills that lengthen a muscle and then flex it. A rubberband-like response that the muscle undergoes where it's stretched beyond normal resting length, then quickly contracted.

power ball *See* medicine ball.

power chain Flexing one muscle and then another, and still another in perfect synchrony.

progressive overload Gradually increasing the intensity of a workout.

protein Essential element of some foods, used by the body to build and maintain muscles, manufacture red blood cells, produce hormones, boost the immune system, and keep hair, fingernails, and skin healthy.

quadratus lomborum Lower back muscles important in spine stability.

quadriceps The muscles on the front of the thigh, consisting of the rectus femoris, vastus lateralis, vastus medialis, and vastus intermedius.

reaction time   The amount of time from when an individual thinks about initiating a movement until when muscles actually take action.

rectus abdominis   A long strap-like muscle extending from the lower-middle ribcage to the pubis.

repetitions (reps)   The number of times you perform a specific exercise.

rhomboids   The muscles between the shoulder blades that are used to keep the shoulders back.

rotator cuff   Four muscles—the supraspinatus, infraspinatus, teres minor, and subscapularis—that rotate the arm.

round   A time period, generally 3 minutes, during fitness boxing.

saturated fats   Fatty acids, abundant in red meat, lard, butter, hard cheeses, and some vegetable oils (palm, coconut, and cocoa butter) and partially hydrogenated oils. Each molecule carries the maximum amount of hydrogen atoms. These fats will solidify at room temperature.

scapulae   The shoulder blades.

shadowboxing   Using combination punches against an imaginary opponent, emphasizing footwork, defense, and correct form.

slip   Tilting the upper body out of the way of a punch.

soft   Maintaining a slight bend in your elbows and knees.

soleus   The muscle underneath the calf muscle. It adds volume to the lower leg.

speed bag   A small air-filled bag attached to the ceiling used by boxers to improve the speed and rhythm of their punches.

stability ball   A round or peanut-shaped ball used to perform exercises on to improve strength, flexibility, and balance.

static stretching   Holding a stretch at a point of tension.

steady state   Moving at a comfortable but challenging pace.

super-slow training   Performing a set of exercises where each repetition may last from 4 to 10 seconds.

sympathetic nervous system (SNS)   One of two divisions of the autonomic nervous system, the SNS prepares the body for action. It tends to speed up the body's systems.

tendon   Fibrous cord-like connective tissue that connects muscle to bone.

trans fatty acid   Usually found in margarine, this is a fatty acid that has been hydrogenated.

transverse abdominis   A flat girdle-like muscle underneath the obliques and rectus abdominis.

trapezius   The muscles on the upper shoulder beside the neck.

triceps   The muscles in the back of the upper arm.

unsaturated fats   Fatty acids in which some of the hydrogen atoms in each molecule have been replaced by double bonds.

uppercut   An upthrusting boxing move that keeps the elbow bent at 90 degrees throughout the move.

warm up   A gradual increase in the intensity of exercise to increase body temperature, muscle elasticity, and contractility.

wind sprints   Moving faster than normal during activity so that you feel winded.

Resources

On the Web

The following sites offer more information about boxing in general, and some information about fitness boxing:

www.balazsboxing.com

www.ekickboxing.com

www.goaero.com

www.ringside.com

www.rossboxing.com

These sites are good sources for buying fitness boxing equipment:

www.centuryfitness.com

www.everlastboxing.com

www.macho.com

www.performbetter.com

www.power-systems.com

www.spriproducts.com

www.titleboxing.com

Books, Magazines, and Newsletters

The following books are good sources for general health, nutrition, and wellness information:

Benson, Herbert. *The Wellness Book.* New York: Simon & Schuster, 1993.

Coleman, Ellen. *Eating for Endurance.* Palo Alto, California: Bull Publishing, 1992.

McArdle, William D., Frank I. Katch, and Victor L. Katch. *Exercise Physiology— Energy, Nutrition, and Human Performance, Sixth Edition.* Philadelphia: Lippincott, Williams & Wilkins, 2006.

Seabourne, T.G. *The Martial Arts Athlete— Mental and Physical Conditioning for Peak Performance.* Boston: YMAA Publication Center, 1998.

Weatherwax, Dawn, and Sonia Weiss. *The Complete Idiot's Guide to Sports Nutrition.* Indianapolis: Alpha Books, 2003.

Wilmore, J., and D. Costill. *Physiology of Sport and Exercise.* Champaign, Illinois: Human Kinetics Publishers, 2004.

Health and fitness information changes almost monthly. Keep up with the latest trends by reading the following magazines and newsletters:

Fitness

Men's Fitness

Men's Health

Muscle & Fitness Hers

Women's Health

Dr. Andrew Weil's Self Healing (available at www.drweilselfhealing.com)

Shape

Index

C

D

G

H

T

Check Out These
Best-Sellers

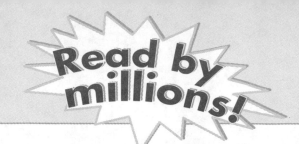

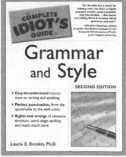

Grammar and Style
SECOND EDITION

- Easy-to-understand instructions on writing and speaking
- Perfect punctuation, from the apostrophe to the semi-colon
- Rights and wrongs of sentence structure, word usage, spelling, and much, much more

Laurie E. Rozakis, Ph.D.

1-59257-115-8 • $16.95

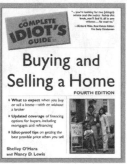

Buying and Selling a Home
FOURTH EDITION

- What to expect when you buy or sell a home—with or without a broker
- Updated coverage of financing options for buyers, including mortgages and refinancing
- Idiot-proof tips on getting the best possible price when you sell

Shelley O'Hara and Nancy D. Lewis

1-59257-120-4 • $18.95

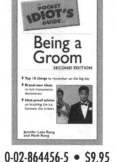

Being a Groom
SECOND EDITION

- Top 10 things to remember on the big day
- Brand-new ideas on hot honeymoon destinations
- Idiot-proof advice on breaking the ice between the in-laws

Jennifer Lata Rung and Mark Rung

0-02-864456-5 • $9.95

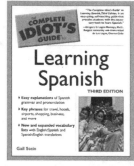

Learning Spanish
THIRD EDITION

- Easy explanations of Spanish grammar and pronunciation
- Key phrases for travel, hotels, airports, shopping, business, and more
- New and expanded vocabulary lists with English/Spanish and Spanish/English translations

Gail Stein

0-02-864451-4 • $18.95

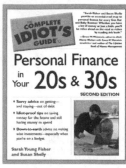

Personal Finance in Your 20s & 30s
SECOND EDITION

- Savvy advice on getting—and staying—out of debt
- Idiot-proof tips on saving money for the future and still having money to spend
- Down-to-earth advice on making wise investments—especially when you're on a budget

Sarah Young Fisher and Susan Shelly

0-02-864374-7 • $19.95

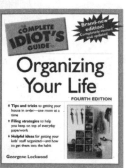

Organizing Your Life
FOURTH EDITION

- Tips and tricks to getting your house in order—one room at a time
- Filing strategies to help you keep on top of everyday paperwork
- Helpful ideas for getting your kids' stuff organized—and how to get them into the habit

Georgene Lockwood

1-59257-413-0 • $16.95

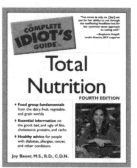

Total Nutrition
FOURTH EDITION

- Food group fundamentals from the dairy, fruit, vegetable, and grain worlds
- Essential information on the good, bad, and ugly of fats, cholesterol, proteins, and carbs
- Healthy advice for people with diabetes, allergies, cancer, and other conditions

Joy Bauer, M.S., R.D., C.D.N.

1-59257-439-4 • $18.95

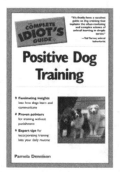

Positive Dog Training

- Fascinating insights into how dogs learn and communicate
- Proven pointers for training without punishment
- Expert tips for incorporating training into your daily routine

Pamela Dennison

0-02-864463-8 • $14.95

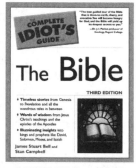

The Bible
THIRD EDITION

- Timeless stories from Genesis to Revelation and all the wondrous tales in between
- Words of wisdom from Jesus Christ's teachings and the episodes of the Apostles
- Illuminating insights into kings and prophets like David, Solomon, Moses, and Isaiah

James Stuart Bell and Stan Campbell

1-59257-389-4 • $18.95

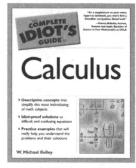

Calculus

- Descriptive concepts that simplify the most intimidating of math subjects
- Idiot-proof solutions to difficult and confusing equations
- Practice examples that will really help you understand the problems and their solutions

W. Michael Kelley

0-02-864365-8 • $18.95

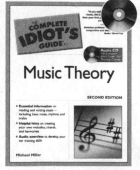

Music Theory
SECOND EDITION

- Essential information on reading and writing music—including basic notes, rhythms, and harmonies
- Helpful hints on creating your own melodies, chords, and harmonies
- Audio exercises to develop your ear training skill

Michael Miller

1-59257-437-8 • $19.95

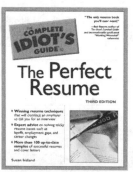

The Perfect Resume
THIRD EDITION

- Winning resume techniques that will convince an employer to call you for an interview
- Expert advice on solving tricky resume issues such as layoffs, employment gaps, and career changes
- More than 100 up-to-date samples of successful resumes and cover letters

Susan Ireland

0-02-864440-9 • $14.95

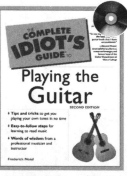

Playing the Guitar
SECOND EDITION

- Tips and tricks to get you playing your own tunes in no time
- Easy-to-follow steps for learning to read music
- Words of wisdom from a professional musician and instructor

Frederick Noad

0-02-864244-9 • $21.95

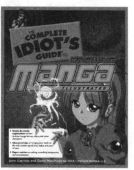

MANGA ILLUSTRATED

- Step-by-step explanations of how to draw manga faces, characters, and color characters
- Whimsical tips on bringing your work to life with modern graphic art, styles, and pops of color
- Expert advice on crafting compelling backgrounds and environments

John Layman and David Manchess for VOLA + DESIGN INDRA S.L.L.

1-59257-335-5 • $19.95

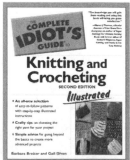

Knitting and Crocheting
SECOND EDITION *Illustrated*

- An all-new selection of easy-to-follow patterns with step-by-step illustrated instructions
- Crafty tips on choosing the right yarn for your project
- Simple advice for going beyond the basics to create more advanced projects

Barbara Breiter and Gail Diven

1-59257-089-5 • $16.95

More than *450 titles* available at
booksellers and online retailers everywhere